The
Ins and Outs
of Gay Sex

A Medical Handbook for Men

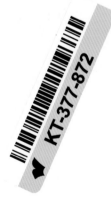

KT-377-872

Stephen E. Goldstone, M.D.

A DELL TRADE PAPERBACK

A DELL TRADE PAPERBACK

Published by
Dell Publishing
a division of
Random House, Inc.
1540 Broadway
New York, New York 10036

Illustrations by Ira C. Smith

Library of Congress Cataloging in Publication Data
Goldstone, Stephen E.
     The ins and outs of gay sex : a medical handbook /
Stephen E. Goldstone.
         p.   cm.
     ISBN 0-440-50846-0
     1. Gay men—Health and hygiene—Handbooks, manuals, etc.
2. Sex instruction for gay men—Handbooks, manuals, etc.
3. Safe sex in AIDS prevention—Handbooks, manuals, etc.
I. Title.
RA777.8.G65   1999
613.9'5'086642—dc21   98-51700
                                                               CIP

Printed in the United States of America

Published simultaneously in Canada

May 1999

10   9   8

RRD

For my two sons and my partner, Bruce Karp.
Together, you have taught me about love and made
my life a joy to live. For that I am truly blessed.

ACKNOWLEDGMENTS

I had been thinking about writing this book for many months, and it might not have come to fruition as quickly had Stanley Siegel and Daniel Wolfe not pushed me to sit down and write the proposal. But their support did not end there. They diligently reviewed what I had written, offered pertinent suggestions that made it better, and then steered me to my agent, Barbara Lowenstein.

I am indebted to Barbara Lowenstein and the staff at Lowenstein and Associates who sold this book before I even knew what had happened.

Overcome with the enormity of this project, I thank Joseph Aversano and Robert Caruso, two of the best friends anyone could hope for, who brought me to the top of a mountain in paradise, where I found the inspiration to write.

As the pages poured out of my computer, I relied upon the members of my writing group, Mark Alpert, Johanna Fiedler, Dave King, Melissa Knox, Eva Meklor, Cheryl Morrison, and David Spears, who helped me eliminate my passive voice, clean up language and sentence structure, and reined me in when I went "over the top." I thank them for learning far more than they wanted or needed to know about gay sex.

I was fortunate to have at my disposal a group of outstanding physicians and physician assistants who willingly answered my questions, filled in gaps in my knowledge, and then offered welcome comments on the manuscript. My thanks go out to Doctors Jeffrey Glick, Robert Gluck, Edward Goldberg, Howard Grossman, Lawrence Hitzeman, Michael Mullen, Michael Swerdlow, and Todd Yancey and physician assistants Russell Chieffe and Florentino Reyes.

I must also offer a special thanks to Dr. Franklin Lowe, a urologist, who let me pick his extremely knowledgeable brain as I wrote the chapters on male genitalia.

I am fortunate to be surrounded by great friends who offered their own personal insights into gay sex, shared their experiences, and willingly read what I had written. They opened my eyes to topics that needed to be covered and dispensed loads of encouragement whenever I got bogged down. Thanks especially to Peter Ezrin, Seth Shulman, Joey Smith, and Ben Stilp.

When I finally turned in the manuscript, I learned how truly lucky I was to have found a wonderful editor in Tom Spain and his assistant, Mitch Hoffman, at Dell. Tom's hard work helped to make this book far better than I could have on my own.

I am forever indebted to my patients, who taught me far more about caregiving than any text or teacher I encountered throughout my career. Their questions and concerns formed the framework of this book. It could not have been written without them.

I must also thank Susan Harper, who kept my office running smoothly and my patients happy while I was busy writing. Ira Smith deserves much credit for his fantastic drawings, which add so much to the text.

I want to thank the very many people who have influenced my life and helped me to grow into the person who could write this book. Catherine Hiller helped me find my "writer's voice," while Dr. Stephen Remen guided me toward self-awareness and, more important, self-acceptance. My parents have always been there for me during the highs and sometime lows of my life, offering encouragement and steadfast assurance of their love.

Every day I am thankful for the boundless love and encouragement I receive from my two sons and my partner, Bruce Karp. This book grew out of his love and support for me.

And last but certainly not least, I am thankful for my two sons and the joy they bring to my life. With each day they continue to surpass my expectations.

I know this list is long, but it had to be, for every one of these people was an integral link in the chain that produced this book. If I've left you out, please accept my apologies, for it was in no way intentional.

CONTENTS

ix

Many of us learn about sex with men in all the wrong places—bars, bathrooms, and backseats—but rarely from anyone who knows what he's talking about. Straight men may turn to their parents or authoritative books for answers, but most gay men would be too embarrassed or even afraid. And if you had the courage to ask parents for help, most, knowing little about gay sexual practices, are ill equipped to provide it.

During my own coming out I attributed every rash, itch, and sore throat I got to my sexual experiences. Before AIDS, I searched bookstores for answers, worried that doing "this" or trying "that" had dealt me a lethal blow. I found how-to books filled with tantalizing pictures, but I already knew how-to. I needed to know what-if. Now, many years later, as I walk through stores, shelves overflow with books on HIV and the joys of gay sex but little has been written about the many other sexually related problems gay men face. Most gay men still don't know the answers to their questions even many years after escaping the closet. And contrary to that popular saying, ignorance is never bliss.

As a physician, every day I see how this dangerous lack of knowledge impacts on our health. Sure, we know about HIV, but what about the more than twenty other sexually transmitted diseases (STDs) infecting over 12 million Americans each year? Although these other STDs may not carry the same grave prognosis as HIV, many are just as incurable and all of them can make you miserable. Day after day men come to my office and ask the same question: "I have safe sex, so how did I get this?" I wrote this book to answer that question.

Most physicians freely admit that they know little about gay sex other than its implication as a cause of AIDS. I recall a young man sitting in my office, having heard rumors that I was definitely gay-friendly and possibly even gay. He came to me as a last resort, having been told by a different surgeon that he required a drastic operation to treat an anal disorder he had ignored for too long. The proposed surgery was so radical that the man's anus might never be normal again. When he asked if he would ever be able to have anal sex again, that surgeon replied, "I hope not. That's what got you into this terrible predicament in the first place."

I wish I could tell you that this story is pure fiction, but it's not. I wish I could tell you that it happened many years ago, in a less enlightened time. Sorry, I heard it only a few weeks ago. I wish I could tell you that the young man came to me from some small town buried deep in the Bible Belt. I can't. He lived less than ten miles outside of a city boasting the largest gay population and possibly the best medical care found in the United States. Sadly, homophobia is rampant in this country, as is a general lack of knowledge about STDs. I wrote this book to help you before and after you see your doctor.

Throughout this book, I've used stories to illustrate key points. Although the names—and sometimes much more—have most definitely been changed to protect the not-so-innocent, they are all based in fact. The word "gay" appears throughout these pages, but the text is meant for all men who have sex with men, no matter how they classify their sexual preference.

Before going forward with this book, prepare yourself for some graphic depictions of diseases, bodily functions, and parts of your male anatomy that may seem far afield from the topic of gay sex. They're not. Sexual gratification is no small feat. It's dependent on a complex chain of events, and understanding how it all fits together can maximize your pleasure and protect you from harm.

I can't promise that, by reading this book, you'll never be treated unfairly by a doctor or healthcare worker, but at least you'll know when you are and what to do about it. I also can't promise that learning from this book will protect you from an STD, but at least you'll enter every sexual relationship armed with enough knowledge to minimize your risk. Know how to make your sex hot, and safe—and not just from HIV.

When I was coming out, no book had the answers I needed, and even today, none is available. That's why I wrote this book for you.

CHAPTER 1

Anal Sex—

OR SO WHAT IF IT'S NOT A VAGINA?

I *shook my head. I still could not find anything wrong. Alex rolled over on the table. Even with the new mustache he still looked like the surfer boy he'd been.*

"What's wrong with me?" he asked.

I rested my hand on his shoulder. "Nothing as far as I can see. You're not too tight."

"I must be. Richard's not that big. I did everything you said and I still can't take him."

"You're tensing up," I said. He tried to argue, but I stopped him. "Not willfully. It's beyond your control. Maybe anal sex isn't for you. There are plenty of other ways to satisfy Richard."

He looked away. "You don't understand. This is important. If I don't do this . . ." His voice trailed off. "Can't you put me to sleep or something? Make it wider?"

"It's wide enough." I gently directed him to look at me. "There is nothing wrong down there. What else is bothering you?"

He didn't answer for several minutes, but I waited. Some things can't be rushed.

Whether we call it anal sex, anal intercourse, or just plain fucking, this type of sex is an integral part of sexual relations

1

for many men who have sex with men. But the practice is in no way limited to gay men; many women enjoy it too. In a recent survey of 100,000 women, *Redbook Magazine* found that 42 percent of women had tried it once, and, for 2 percent, anal sex was an important part of their sexual relationships. We are not alone! Many men enjoy anal sex; the experience is pleasurable and vital to their sex life.

I remember standing in horror as a physician I worked with berated a gay man he treated with a terse "Your asshole is for shitting, not fucking!" Well, this is not the case. Anal sex can be both pleasurable and safe if practiced properly. Unfortunately, homophobia has clouded the issue. Ignorance and rumor often magnify our fears about possible injury. Many gay men refuse to discuss anal sex with their physicians, and most physicians know little if anything about it—other than that it transmits HIV.

Many women view vaginal intercourse as the major step in their sexual evolution, giving considerable thought to who will be their first. Men joke about losing their virginity after their first anal sex experience and minimize its significance. True, we don't have a hymen to rupture, but anal sex is not an insignificant step, emotionally or physically. Many men view anal sex as the final step on their path to gayness. (Once you've done it you *must* be gay.) For some it's a sign of their first true love. Others view anal sex as an assault on their masculinity. Unfortunately, some men recall their first episode of anal sex as the horror of sexual abuse, and they may never recover. In any case, you shouldn't bend over for anyone until you're ready.

Physiologically, anal sex must not be taken lightly. Sure, you can't get pregnant, but there are a million other things you can get instead. Anal sex is probably the highest-risk sexual act performed by men who have sex with men—and not just because of HIV. Most sexually transmitted diseases (STDs) pass between partners during anal sex—even without ejaculation. And a condom may not be protection enough. In this era of sexual freedom, it is almost impossible to have a healthy sex life and avoid an STD. Before you let that guy inside you, make sure he's clean and you're protected.

If you have anal sex regularly, use these pages as a guide; they may protect you from injury and STDs. And for those of you who aren't ready for anal sex, read on. Someday a relationship might arise when it becomes something that you both desire.

Anatomy

Anal intercourse differs from vaginal intercourse in several significant ways. First and foremost, a hole is not just a hole, and a woman's vagina is anatomically very different from your anus. The colon's purpose, as we all know, is to transport digestive waste from your small intestine to your anal opening where it's excreted. As part of this task, the colon's lining, or mucosa, is specially equipped to absorb water from the liquid waste of your small intestines and turn it into solid feces. When your colonic mucosa doesn't work properly, diarrhea results. Your colon's heightened absorption capability makes it a particularly susceptible entryway for many infections; HIV, of course, is one of the most deadly.

Your colon is approximately six feet long, and unless your partner is something of a "giant" among men, anal intercourse affects only the last few inches. This area includes your anus and rectum; although they both are regions of your colon, they are, in actuality, two very distinct anatomic sites. Your anus is lined by squamous cells, which are closely related to skin. Your rectum resembles the rest of your colon. Importantly, your anus has nerve endings capable of experiencing pain while your rectum does not.

The muscles that control bowel movements, or sphincters, as they are commonly called, are concentrated in your anus and lower rectum. These muscles can be divided into an external sphincter and internal sphincter. (See Figure 1.1.) Your external sphincter, the outermost band of muscle, is under your direct control. You can willfully tighten it to keep gas or feces from leaking out, and you can relax it for defecation. Your internal sphincter muscle abuts your colon wall. It is an involuntary muscle, and as such you cannot willfully cause it to relax or contract. When feces enter your lower rectum, the internal sphincter involuntarily relaxes for defecation. If you're miles from a bathroom or in the middle of some speech, you depend on your external sphincter to contract and prevent an embarrassing situation from occurring. The rectal wall also contains nerve fibers that tell you the difference between feces and gas.

Just as your internal sphincter muscle involuntarily relaxes when feces enter your rectum, it *involuntarily* contracts when a penis or other object attempts to enter from the outside. As the word "involuntarily" implies, this sphincter contraction is beyond your ability to control, no matter how relaxed or sexually aroused you are. The relaxation and contraction of the internal sphincter allows you to pass large bowel movements painlessly, yet a penis of equal or smaller size can hurt during insertion. An anal tear can occur during the initial phase of anal sex precisely because your partner pushes his penis through your closed sphincter. Think of his penis as a battering ram, one for which your internal sphincter is no match.

Hygiene

Before moving on, I must write a few words about hygiene. Most men who enjoy anal sex or anal stimulation are

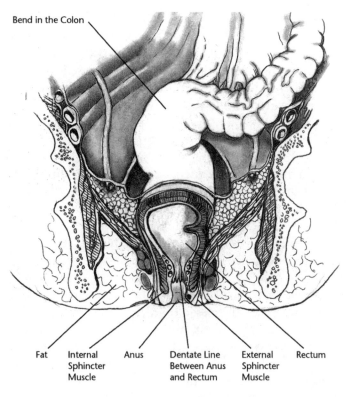

Bend in the Colon

Fat | Internal Sphincter Muscle | Anus | Dentate Line Between Anus and Rectum | External Sphincter Muscle | Rectum

Figure 1.1: Normal Anatomy

fastidious about keeping this area clean, and, in fact, they can be *too* fastidious. I remember a patient who came to me for treatment of pain and bleeding with his bowel movements. When I examined him, I noticed deep cuts in the skin surrounding his anus. Upon questioning, I discovered that he wiped so hard with toilet paper to get clean before anal sex that he was quite literally wiping away his skin. Well, I am sorry to report that no matter how hard you try, an anus is still an anus, and it will never be the silk purse you've dreamed of. Before sex, I recommend that you gently wipe away any fecal residue from your outer skin with a moist tissue. Wet cotton balls or Tucks do an excellent job, but stay away from those baby-wipe–type towels. Most contain perfumes that can irritate your sensitive skin.

An enema or douching prior to sex is not advised, as this can force a large volume of fluid into your rectum, which you may not fully evacuate before sex. The in-and-out motion of your partner's penis or fingers stimulates colonic contractions, and any residual enema will spill out, creating more of a mess. Chronic enema use also can produce severe constipation. In worst cases, men become so dependent on enemas that they cannot move their bowels without them.

If you worry that feces remain in your colon and you cannot have a bowel movement before sex, try a gentle wash-out with an ear syringe. (When you were a baby, your mother used them to clean your ears, but now that you're a big boy . . .) Ear syringes, available in most pharmacies, come in two styles: a blunt, wide tip meant only to cover the hole in your ear, and a slender, tapered style for insertion into your ear canal. Be sure to purchase the slender, tapered style and fill it with warm water. Lubricate the tip, insert it into your rectum, and gently squeeze the bulb several times. This will instill much less liquid than an enema. Also, you are more likely to expel the water and any fecal residue fully.

Foreplay

Foreplay is as important in anal sex as it is in vaginal intercourse. Although your anus does not self-lubricate as a vagina does during foreplay, this stage is critical if you want to achieve eventual sphincter relaxation. It also helps you judge whether your partner will follow your wishes. For penetration to occur without injury, your partner must wait until you are able to receive. Most injuries during anal sex occur when penetration is rushed or when the receiving partner has not consented or is not relaxed.

You must incorporate safe-sex practices into your foreplay. In other words, condoms are not just for fucking. Quite often during foreplay your partner rubs his penis against your buttocks and anal opening. Although HIV is rarely spread without ejaculation, it can be. (Pre-cum carries HIV and can seep inside.) Moreover, numerous other infections, including herpes, anal warts, molluscum, and syphilis, can spread between partners from rubbing without penetration. You can catch most of these nasties with skin-to-skin contact alone. (See Chapters 3 and 4.) And although these infections are not lethal, they can make you miserable and may be incurable. Therefore, place a condom on your partner's penis as soon as you anticipate any contact with your anal area. If he complains, remind him that infections travel both ways. You're protecting him from anything you might be carrying.

Pleasure awaits when you stimulate the many nerve endings buried in your anal skin. Some men enjoy light rubbing, while others prefer a heavier touch. Avoid anything that can tear or cut the skin, because feces contain many bacteria that can easily infect a wound. Touching the anus during foreplay is purely for pleasure's sake. Although it may heighten desire for anal sex, it does not cause lubrication or direct relaxation of the sphincter. In fact, the sphincter responds by twitching closed momentarily with each touch. Some men enjoy anilingus as another way to stimulate their partners, but beware of STDs. (See Chapter 9.)

Many men insert fingers or sex toys into their anus as part of foreplay or masturbation, but this is not without risk. Fingers can be more dangerous than a partner's penis if sharp nails, dangling cuticles, diamond rings (you get the idea) cut the delicate lining of the anus. Men with HIV need to pay particular attention to anal hygiene and avoid injury, because their ability to fight infection is impaired. Your rectum lacks nerves responsive to touch, so most tactile pleasure comes from rubbing your anus and surrounding skin, not from penetration. Penetration stimulates pelvic muscle contractions, which can heighten an orgasm.

Before inserting a finger into your anus, be sure that your nails (or your partner's) are free of sharp or jagged edges and cuts that transmit infection. Remember: Any cut on a finger also can become infected with bacteria normally present in the anus. A latex glove or finger cot helps protect you from your partner's fingers acting as a conduit for STDs. (See Chapters 3 and 4.) Do not insert more than one finger into your anus to stretch it in anticipation of anal sex. Stretching with several fingers can cause a dangerous tear and plunge your sphincter into painful spasm, which will prevent penetration. Sphincter injury may weaken the muscle so that it cannot contract adequately. Loss of bowel control may result.

Toys

He was waiting for me when I arrived at my office first thing Monday morning. Dressed in his navy pinstripe suit and white starched shirt, not a hair out of place and a leather briefcase at his side, he looked every bit the corporate attorney. "What's the problem?" I asked, but he didn't answer. "I can't help you if I don't know what's wrong."

"Didn't Dr. Gordon tell you?" he asked. I shook my head. "Well, there was a lot of traffic coming home from the country. . . ."

I could not understand what traffic had to do with his visit, but I could wait. "Go on," I prompted.

"Chuck and I were bored, so we pulled over at one of those roadside stands. . . . We bought a zucchini and some Crisco."

I was beginning to understand. "You did this while you were driving?"

He nodded. "We weren't going very fast. When Chuck had to change lanes . . . it sort of got away. It won't come out."

If you enjoy sex toys or dildos, don't pass them back and forth between you and your partner unless they're covered in a condom that is changed between each insertion. Avoid toys with sharp or pointed edges; instead use ones with tapered ends. Your rectal canal is not a straight line; rather, it curves back toward your tailbone. Thus, insertion of any object should be directed a little posterior (toward your back) and not toward the front.

Approximately eight inches from the anal opening, the colon takes a sharp turn to the left. You must know this if you insert a long object into your rectum. Stiff dildos or other objects may not be able to negotiate the turn and may pass right through your colon wall. A colon rupture is a surgical emergency, because bacteria can spread quickly throughout your abdomen or pelvis. When shopping for a new toy, choose one made of soft latex. Harder materials are less giving (and forgiving) and offer greater risk of rupturing your colon.

Besides choosing a soft dildo or sex toy, find one with a blunt, tapered end so that your sphincter gradually stretches as penetration occurs. A wide base or flange at the opposite end prevents its escape into your rectum if you lose your grip. (Toys can become quite slippery.) Should this occur, your sphincter will close. Don't try to "dig" the object out. (You aren't drilling for oil.) Most often you'll pass it like a bowel movement if you squat down and wait. If it's still inside after an hour, see a doctor. Failure to remove a foreign object can lead to colon perforation. Attempts to wash it out with enemas or a shower spray (as my patient did) will only push it farther up into the colon. Usually a doctor can retrieve it in his office or an emergency room with special instruments. In extreme circumstances, a trip to the operating room with anesthesia may be necessary, but only to dilate your rectum so the toy can be grabbed. Horror stories of men needing extensive abdominal surgery usually are not based in fact—unless they have ruptured their colon.

As always, common sense is the rule. Learn to be sensitive with your hand when inserting anything into your rectum. If there is any resistance or pain, change the angle of penetration or pull it out. *Never* persist. Communicate any discomfort to your partner, and be sure he is responsive to your complaints.

Anal Sex Technique

With a little understanding of physiology, anal intercourse can be performed safely. Like any muscle, your internal sphincter can contract for only so long before it fatigues and must relax. When it relaxes, your partner can safely insert his penis without causing you pain. How do you make your muscle fatigue? Easy. Unroll a latex condom over your partner's penis. Natural-membrane condoms don't protect you from HIV, and ultra-sheer styles can break during sex. Lubricate the condom well with a water-soluble solution (Eros, Foreplay, and Wet are just a few of the available brands), because it won't harm latex condoms, and it is readily broken down by your body after intercourse. Besides weakening condoms, oil-based lubricants occlude your very sensitive anal glands and can cause infection. Read labels carefully before buying. Many lubricants, including Elbow Grease and hand creams, are oil based. The lubricant is very important; don't trust the choice to a partner grabbing whatever is handy from his nightstand. Many lubricants (even water-soluble ones) contain dyes and perfumes that can be especially irritating to your sensitive skin and anal lining. I have seen men who developed terrible skin allergies and colitis from lubricants. So find a brand you like, but remember that what works for you may not work for your partner.

Apply a generous amount of lubricant to your outer anal area. Inserting fingers into your anus may cause tearing and is not necessary if you thoroughly coat your partner. A well-lubricated penis may be less traumatic than a finger with sharp nails. Gently lower yourself onto your partner's penis to the point where you feel discomfort. (See Figure 1.2.) This corresponds to the moment when his penis begins to stretch your contracted internal sphincter muscle. Stay in this same position, with your partner's penis applying constant and gentle pressure against your internal sphincter muscle. His pressure will cause your muscle to maintain its contraction until it tires and must relax. And no, you won't be suspended over him in a fit of anticipation for hours upon hours. Thankfully, the muscle usually tires within thirty to sixty seconds. When you feel your sphincter relax, sit the rest of the way down on his penis. After a couple of up-and-down movements, your muscle will be sufficiently stretched so that you can move to any position you like.

It is also important that you do not stimulate your penis (manually or orally) while your partner attempts penetration. Stimulation immediately causes your sphincter muscles to contract and only increases the time it takes your sphincter to relax. Of course, once you accommodate your partner, stimulate all you want.

I recommend that anal intercourse be initiated with the receptive partner on top, because this position allows him to be in control. When you are on top, you control penetration according to when your muscle contracts and when it relaxes. Injury occurs from persistent insertion through a

Gently lower yourself onto your partner until you feel pain. Stop and wait for your sphincter to relax and then sit the rest of the way down.

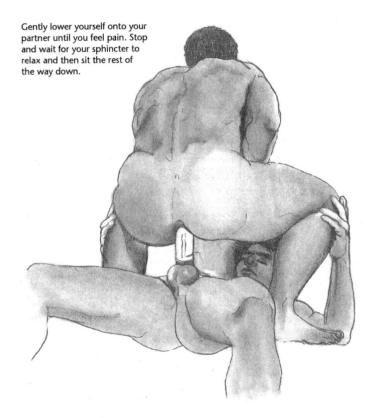

Figure 1.2: Anal Sex

tight anus. If your partner is on top and he feels your internal sphincter tighten, he will naturally push harder because he wants to be inside. Your sphincter is no match for his desire.

If insertion causes you pain, then his penis must be withdrawn and your muscle allowed to rest before any further attempts are made. Often intense pain means your muscle has gone into spasm (abnormally tight contraction), and it may be anywhere from hours to days before it relaxes again.

Persistent insertion through a closed muscle can tear your anal canal (cause a fissure) or rupture your sphincter. (See Chapter 2.) Blood may or may not be present, and you might require medical attention. For anoreceptive intercourse to be safe, it must be pain free.

Since most of us are size queens, patients often ask what they should do to accommodate an unusually large penis. Well, occasionally you can't. And again I advise common sense: If it hurts, don't do it. But try we must, so here are some easy rules to follow. First and foremost, your partner's length is not usually the problem, but his girth may be. Your rectum is long enough to accommodate just about any penis, but it may not be able to stretch comfortably to accommodate his width. Once his penis gets past your sphincter muscles (about three inches into your rectum), you're usually home free. Even if he gets thicker at the base, your buttocks keep you from descending all the way down on him. Again, I don't advise multiple-finger insertion as a means to "predilate" your sphincter because you can end up with a nasty tear. Rectal dilators, sold in surgical supply stores, typically come in a set of four graduated sizes (diameter, not length). They are blunt tipped for easy insertion. Lie on your side and start with the smallest one (usually smaller than your finger). Lubricate it well with a water-soluble solution and insert it by applying gentle, constant pressure against your opening until you feel your sphincter relax. Then push it the rest of the way in. Leave it in for about five minutes and then, if you're up to it, progress to the next-larger size until you've used all four. This provides you with a stepwise sphincter dilation so that, it's hoped, you can accommodate your partner. Incorporate these dilators into foreplay, working up to the largest size before your partner attempts penetration. If you use them hours before a date, your sphincter may regain its strength before you climb into bed. Don't worry about needing the dilators forever. Once you can take your partner, you probably won't need the dilators any longer—or at least not until your next boyfriend. Inserting dilators can be a real turn-on for a partner. If he wants to help, that's fine, as long as he lets you guide him. You don't want him ramming the dilator in before you're ready.

If you feel very tight—perhaps you never had anal sex before, had recent anal surgery, or are frightened from previous bad experiences—you will need to take more time. Dilators are also very helpful for men in this situation, but instead of rapidly moving up from smallest to largest size, use one dilator (start with the smallest) for ten minutes three times a day. And no, you don't have to do it on your lunch break. Try it once in the morning before work, after work, and before bed. Each week progress to the next-larger size. It will take a month, but in the end you'll be rewarded.

Expect more difficulty and discomfort if you have a very tight sphincter. If it hurts when you first get the dilator in, don't pull it out. That will only further aggravate your muscle spasm. Wait ten minutes. By then your sphincter will have relaxed and pulling it out should be easy. If you do have pain, ask your doctor for a mild topical anesthetic to coat the dilator. Once it's in, the medicine will numb your sphincter. Don't use an anesthetic for anal sex, because it decreases sensations and you won't experience as much pleasure from anoreceptive intercourse as you otherwise would have.

What do you do if the dilators are still not big enough? Thank the Lord for your good fortune, and then ask for the next-larger set. Dilators come in many graduated sizes, and you should be able to find some that will approximate your partner.

I am often asked if a dildo is just as good. Many men find them more arousing and prefer the soft feel of latex to the hard plastic of most dilators. The answer is an equivocal maybe, and again, common sense applies. If you have a scar from surgery that you are trying to stretch, you may need the firmer plastic or a medical dilator. Men tend to buy large dildos, but if it's almost as large as or larger than your partner, it can cause as much damage as he can. Start out with something small, midway between your finger and your partner, that you can accommodate without much difficulty. You want muscle relaxation without spasm. I also prefer the graduated sizes provided by medical dilators. Unless you buy several dildos, this benefit of progressive dilatation won't happen with a single dildo. As with a penis, coat your dildo with a water-soluble lubricant.

What if all this fails, and you still cannot accommodate your partner? Well, I'm sorry to report that occasionally anal intercourse is impossible. For gay men, anoreceptive intercourse is steeped in psychological overtones, and limitations other than physical may prevent penetration. I have had couples in my office pleading to "make him relax so we can fuck." Many times the couple is talking to a surgeon when they should be talking to a therapist. With patience, a gentle approach, and counseling, you may be able to overcome the problem.

Just a word about positions. Be creative, and as long as it gets in and doesn't hurt, it's fine. Once you relax and your sphincter accommodates your partner, move to any position you choose. Medically speaking, if you are prone to rectal problems such as hemorrhoids, then a position with your face down puts less pressure on your anal area. When you're on your back with your legs in the air, your hemorrhoids may swell with blood and bleed. You may be able to relax your sphincter better in certain positions, while others may afford deeper penetration. Experimentation is not only fun, it helps you find the optimal position for both you and your partner's enjoyment.

A Word for You Tops

I know you've read it already, but it's so important you're going to read it again: *Your partner must be in control.* Your penis can hurt him seriously if he isn't ready to take it. Foreplay is great. While it may heighten his desire for anal sex, physiologically it doesn't do anything to relax his sphincter. So when you're ready to put it in, do whatever he asks. If he wants you to wait or take it out, listen to him. By persisting, you'll cause more damage, and he may never let you back in again. Many men, even with proper sphincter relaxation, still experience some pain when you first get all the way in. Some find it tolerable, while others will ask you to pull out and let them rest. Your penis has just acted like a dilator, and coming out prevents his sphincter from going into spasm. No doubt he'll let you back in, and because his muscle is already stretched, you'll both have an easier and more enjoyable time.

If your penis is especially long, you may come to a point in penetration that gives your partner pain. Your partner feels the head of your penis stretching the curve in his colon. While you probably won't push through, you can injure him and cause bleeding. If those last few inches make him uncomfortable, hold back.

Always use a condom. STDs pass both ways, and an anus is the highest-risk place for STDs. He can easily infect you with anything lurking in and around his anus. I caution you to assess your risk of catching something from each new partner before sticking it in. You may decide that something less risky (masturbation or even oral sex) might be a wiser choice. (See Chapter 10.) Some men abandon condoms if both partners are HIV positive. Again, I strongly advise against this. There are plenty of other STDs to catch that you may not already have. By not using a condom you also increase your chances of picking up a more resistant strain of HIV than what you already have. (See Chapter 5.)

As soon as you ejaculate, withdraw your penis while keeping a firm grip on the end of the condom. If you wait to pull out, you will start to lose your erection and semen can seep through gaps in the condom at the base of your shaft. This allows STDs out or in, depending on who has what. By holding on to the condom as you withdraw, you prevent it from being left inside.

What if your partner says no to anal sex? That is always his prerogative. Certainly talk about it, exploring feelings as you try to discover reasons for his objection. If he says it hurts, try a course of dilators. Always be mindful of nonverbal cues. (Gritting his teeth while you're poised to enter is not a good sign.) He may be afraid to tell you he doesn't want to do it, and persisting can ruin a good relationship. If he refuses, find other ways to satisfy yourself or move on. If the relationship is important, sex therapy and couples therapy are often beneficial and may solve your problem.

And last, just because you're the top doesn't mean that someday your partner won't ask you to be the bottom. Again, you can always refuse, but you might just like it.

Complications

Gay men who practice anal sex or stimulation tend to assume erroneously that all anal-related problems are caused by their sexual practices. This could not be further from the truth. (See Chapter 2.) If you do develop an anorectal problem, I urge you to contact your physician, for although it may be related to sex, it probably isn't. Besides mentioning your symptoms, tell your doctor that you've had anal sex. If you cannot admit this without embarrassment, find a different doctor!

There are numerous, though thankfully infrequent, complications related to anal sex, but most are infectious and will be covered in subsequent chapters. (See Chapters

2, 3, and 5.) Several complications do need to be discussed now.

BLEEDING Bleeding is probably the most common complication you'll experience during or after anal intercourse. Of course, if you notice it during sex, your partner should immediately withdraw his penis and terminate intercourse. Bleeding also occurs prior to anal sex from finger manipulation, and anal sex should not be attempted until you heal. Painless bleeding most often results from hemorrhoid trauma (see Chapter 2) and stops on its own. Most men know if they have hemorrhoids, but if your bleeding persists for more than a day, see your physician. Bleeding associated with pain is more significant and usually signifies a tear (fissure) in the lining of your anus. (See Chapter 2.) This tear usually sends your sphincter into spasm, which may not subside until the fissure heals fully. Persisting in anal sex can deepen the tear, causing injury to your sphincter muscle. Fortunately, tears usually heal on their own with stool softeners (medications that lubricate your stool for easy passage) and temporary abstinence from anal sex.

PAIN Pain is a very nonspecific symptom after anal sex and is often the first sign of infection (most notably herpes and gonorrhea). Typically, pain begins a few days after intercourse, once the infection has had time to incubate and take hold. Although you may notice a discharge or blisters around your anal opening, most often you will notice nothing at all. (See Chapters 3 and 4.)

Severe pain, with or without bleeding, during intercourse or immediately after may signify damage to your sphincter muscles. These muscles can tear when stretched too much or too quickly. Injured muscle bleeds, but the blood can remain trapped where you won't see it. Instead, you might notice swelling and pressure accompanying the pain—similar to a bruise from a torn muscle in any other part of your body. Treatment includes muscle relaxants, pain relievers, stool softeners, and sitz baths (bathing the area in warm water). Although most muscle injuries are minor and resolve without long-term complications, some doctors believe they weaken the sphincter muscles. Repeated injuries cause cumulative damage and, in later life, may lead to incontinence (an inability to control your bowel movements or gas).

As with all aspects of anal sex, the common-sense rule again applies. If your partner pounds you senseless, then trauma and bleeding are more likely to occur. It is understandable that when you make the decision to have anal sex, your state of sexual arousal is at a feverish pitch. You may have sex several times in a night, and as we all know, the more often you come, the longer it takes to come again. Your partner's constant pounding places your anal canal at a greater risk for injury, and you should stop the moment sex ceases to be pleasurable. Drug use also increases the risks associated with anal sex. Drugs dull sensation, so something that should hurt doesn't. They further increase danger by distorting judgment and allowing you to have sex in ways you ordinarily wouldn't. Drug use fosters unsafe sex. (See Chapter 11.)

PERFORATION *By the time his friend brought him to the emergency room, he could no longer stand. His pulse raced over 100 and his blood pressure barely hit 80. His skin burned with fever and the slightest touch to his abdomen made him scream. An older man probably would have been dead by now; only his youth had kept him alive this long. "What happened?" I asked.*

His lips were dry and his voice faint as he spoke. "I fell off a ladder and landed on a broom. It went up my butt."

Now I'd heard everything. "Did someone do this to you?" I

asked. He shook his head. Even with his body overrun with infection, he wouldn't tell the truth. "How long ago did this happen?"
"Three days."

Although a total (transmural) perforation of your anus or rectum is possible during anal sex, thankfully it is quite rare. Perforation, however, is much more frequent when hands (fisting) or sex toys are inserted into the rectum. These objects tend to be longer, thicker, and less pliable than a penis. If perforation occurs, pain usually is the first symptom. Although it begins immediately, you might barely notice it. The pain progressively worsens as you notice other hallmarks of infection: fever, swelling, and reddening of your buttocks. If the perforation is high up in your rectum, a deadly complication, your buttocks may look normal, and pain, fever, and a sense of pelvic pressure are the only signs. Most often neither you nor your physician can see the actual hole or holes. Typically they are quite small and hidden in the myriad folds in the normal colon lining.

Treatment of a transmural perforation often requires emergency hospitalization, intravenous antibiotics, and surgery to clean out the infection. Unfortunately, most men delay treatment for many reasons: embarrassment, an unwillingness to discuss the problem with their doctor, and/or the unrealistic hope that it will go away on its own. This is an extremely dangerous course to follow as the colon is filled with deadly bacteria that can cause devastating infection once they escape the colon. In extreme situations, ignoring the signs and symptoms of a perforation can cause a colostomy to be needed until the infection heals.

INCONTINENCE Incontinence is the medical term for the inability to control either feces or gas. Doctors describe many degrees of incontinence. In its mildest form, it can be an inability to control gas (which everyone seems to complain of) or a sense of urgency to move your bowels. You feel that if you don't get to a bathroom immediately, you'll soil yourself. In severe cases, people lack the ability to sense stool in their rectum and cannot prevent it from escaping. Clearly, an inability to control gas is more embarrassing than debilitating; complete fecal incontinence, however, can be quite devastating. It requires significant lifestyle changes: a diaper and occasionally a colostomy.

Most people experience episodes of fecal incontinence at some point in their lives, typically during severe bouts of diarrhea. You can't control the diarrhea because your sphincter muscles are not strong enough to hold back the sheer volume of liquid or to prevent its watery consistency from slipping out. Although this type of incontinence is normal and infrequent, it presents a problem for HIV-positive men prone to diarrhea or who take diarrhea-inducing medications (which many antiviral drugs are).

In one medical study of men who practiced anoreceptive intercourse, 25 percent reported at least isolated episodes of fecal incontinence. An age-similar group of heterosexual men had only a 3 percent incontinence rate. When the researchers studied patients with AIDS, the incidence of incontinence rose to 50 percent and probably resulted from a higher rate of frequent loose bowel movements in these individuals.

What does this mean to men who enjoy anal sex? Although the threat of incontinence is small, it is present nonetheless. Incontinence in men who practice anal sex is thought to result from repeated injury to their internal spincter muscle, not the external sphincter, which comes under their voluntary control. Again, although a penis is often the size of a large bowel movement, your sphincter involuntarily relaxes to allow the bowel movement to pass and your muscle is not injured. Insertion of a penis, however, causes your muscle to contract involuntarily. Repeated insertion through a contracted internal sphincter muscle may cause cumulative damage so that the muscle loses its ability to seal the anorectal canal tightly.

Incontinence from anal sex appears to be rare enough so that you probably won't have a problem if you protect your internal sphincter as described. Incontinence rates do increase in proportion to the number of sexual partners a man has. Whether this implies that sex with many partners causes more frequent sphincter injury over a longer period of time or that men with more partners are prone to rougher sexual practices causing more injury is unknown.

Fisting and insertion of extremely large sex toys into the anus results in a much higher incidence of incontinence and is definitely *not* recommended. Incontinence in men who practice either of these types of sex is thought to result from increased damage to their internal sphincter muscles by the large-diameter object.

Summary

Anal stimulation and sex can be pleasurable and safe if practiced properly. The common-sense rule must be applied at all times: If it hurts, don't do it.

- Listen to your partner. Respect his wishes.
- If it hurts or you notice blood, stop immediately.
- Always use a condom even if only rubbing is anticipated.
- Protect fingers with gloves or finger cots.
- Do not pass sex toys back and forth between partners.
- If complications arise, see an understanding physician.
- Fisting and inserting large toys promote incontinence.

CHAPTER 2

Common Anorectal Disorders—

OR PROBLEMS EVEN

STRAIGHT MEN HAVE

He lay on the emergency room stretcher, his face so pale that it was difficult to tell where the sheet ended and he began. "You're a very lucky man," I said. "Passing out is a very serious problem. It's a good thing your roommate found you."

He looked away and said nothing.

"How long had you been bleeding?" I asked.

He shrugged. "Couple of days, but only when I moved my bowels."

I didn't believe him. He had lost half of his blood, and that didn't happen so quickly, not from hemorrhoids. "You should have seen a doctor the moment it started."

"I told you it wasn't so bad."

I patted his shoulder. Maybe he'd talk later. "I'm admitting you to the hospital so we can watch your blood count. Make sure you don't need a transfusion."

I was almost out of the room when he said, "You're not putting down that I was bleeding from my butt, are you?"

"Rectal bleeding from hemorrhoids. That is your diagnosis. I have to be honest."

He bolted upright. "Insurance forms go to my job. They'll know I'm gay."

At some point in their lives, over 50 percent of all Americans suffer from anorectal disorders. Because far less than half of our nation's population is gay, we can safely conclude that most people with these problems did not get them through sex. When a gay man develops rectal bleeding or pain, he often incorrectly attributes it to anal sex. This is a dangerous assumption, since it often causes men to delay seeking treatment due to embarrassment and/or fear of instant "outing." Anal sex certainly can cause injury, but this is more often the exception than the rule. Let me set the record straight (no pun intended): Straight men have hemorrhoids too. And no, your doctor cannot tell from a simple rectal exam that you've been fucked.

The first sign of an anorectal disorder is often a spot of bright-red blood on the toilet paper or in the bowl after a bowel movement. The bleeding may or may not be associated with pain. The entire bowl can even turn red. Although frightening, this does *not* mean that you are hemorrhaging to death. It takes only two drops of blood to turn all the water red. If you see red water, place a tissue against your anus and be sure that the blood keeps dripping before you play drama queen and call for an ambulance. In most cases, after your bowel movement has passed, your anus contracts and creates enough pressure to stop any bleeding. If you follow the simple guidelines set forth in this chapter, most minor anorectal problems can be treated at home without a physician. Of course, if your symptoms do not resolve in a day or two, if they worsen, or if other troubling signs, such as fever or purulent (infected-looking) discharge, arise, seek medical attention immediately.

Hemorrhoids

Millions of years ago humans began to walk upright . . . and got hemorrhoids. A slight exaggeration? Perhaps, but they are mentioned as far back as the Bible and in ancient Greek writings. Many scholars believe that Alexander the Great suffered from hemorrhoids (and also that he was gay, but we won't go there). Napoleon had them and so did President Jimmy Carter. Although Hippocrates performed a hemorrhoidectomy more than 2,000 years ago, most often surgery can be avoided.

Essentially hemorrhoids are varicose veins of the anus and rectum. Hemorrhoids begin as normal veins present at the end of the rectal canal that act as cushions to ease the passage of stool. When these small veins become abnormally dilated, hemorrhoids form. Hemorrhoids are divided into two types: internal and external. (See Figure 2.1.)

Internal hemorrhoids originate inside the rectum and are covered by the colon lining (mucosa). As they enlarge, they

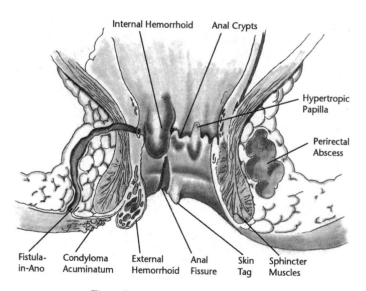

Figure 2.1: Benign Anorectal Disorders

can prolapse (hang) out of the anal opening. When they stick out, they resemble small cherries.

External hemorrhoids, on the other hand, are enlarged veins covered with skin originating in and around the anus. They are always on the outside, and although you may be tempted, they should not be pushed in. Most people have a combination of both types of hemorrhoids: an external component covered with skin leading into the internal portion covered with colonic mucosa.

External hemorrhoids create intense pain when they swell because of nerve irritation in their outer skin covering. The swelling results when blood that normally flows through these veins clots inside them. When blood clots, it causes intense inflammation, and you feel a swollen, hard, and very tender lump just beside your anus. If you bend over far enough and get a good look at your hemorrhoid, it usually looks like a concord grape. Its blue color results from the blood clot within the vein.

You may be wondering how you can see your hemorrhoids or anything else that is bothering you "back there." Of course, it is best to have a physician or partner look, but if you are too embarrassed, try a mirror. Place the mirror on the floor between your feet. Squat down over it in a well-lighted area and gently spread your buttocks. Usually you'll have to place your fingers quite close to your opening to spread your cheeks far enough apart for a close look. Often hemorrhoids will look much smaller than they feel.

Thrombosed (clotted) external hemorrhoids do not bleed unless the clot causes so much pressure that it breaks through the skin. Although this sounds frightening, the bleeding is usually minimal and actually represents the body's own attempt at healing itself by extruding the clot. Once the clot passes, swelling subsides and so does pain. If the clot does not push through the skin, the body slowly dissolves it and reabsorbs the clot back into your bloodstream. As more and more of the clot is reabsorbed, swelling and tenderness decrease. Whether the clot is pushed out or dissolved, usually an external hemorrhoid is history within two to three weeks. All that remains of this painful episode is a fleshy piece of skin (anal tag) at your anal opening . . . until it happens again.

When blood clots in a vein, the resulting inflammation leaves behind a damaged vein. So, once you've had a thrombosed hemorrhoid, you are more likely to get it again—and it may be worse the second time around. This is why most physicians advise complete excision (removal) of a thrombosed hemorrhoid as soon as it occurs. Although technically a surgical procedure, most often it is performed right in the doctor's office with local anesthesia. While some pain is associated with any surgery, in this instance the pain usually is less than what you experienced from the thrombosed hemorrhoid.

In the past, treatment of thrombosed hemorrhoids involved making a small incision into the hemorrhoid and removing the clot. You may encounter a physician today who still recommends this "old" form of therapy, but I advise against it, because a simple "incision and drainage" does not remove the diseased veins, only the clot. Although you will certainly feel better after the clot is removed, your chance of a recurrence is very great. Most surgeons now recommend a complete removal of a hemorrhoid the first time a thrombosis occurs.

Men often wonder why they developed a thrombosed hemorrhoid in the first place. It occurs when normal blood flow through a vein becomes disturbed and begins to clot. Although anal sex can cause clotting, it is not likely to be the cause. Most often hemorrhoids result from bearing down to lift something heavy or pushing out a hard bowel movement. Occasionally something as simple as a cough or sneeze will do it. In most instances you will never know why you got the hemorrhoid.

Although internal hemorrhoids often have an associated external component, they are very different from each other. Internal hemorrhoids are not covered with skin, and as such, they lack nerves that sense pain. While rarely painful, internal hemorrhoids bleed when inflamed. Hard stool rubbing against them creates a tear, or they burst from the pressure of a bowel movement. If you notice painless bleeding after a bowel movement, chances are great that you've got an internal hemorrhoid. Even though painless rectal bleeding is usually from a hemorrhoid, it should never be ignored. I urge you to see a physician if bleeding persists. It can be a symptom of something serious, such as a colon cancer.

In order to prevent hemorrhoids or treat the ones you already have, it is helpful to first understand their causes. Anything that increases pressure in your anorectal canal will predispose you to hemorrhoids. Straining during a bowel movement is the most common cause of increased pressure. When you sit on the toilet and push hard to pass a stool, you force blood into your hemorrhoids and they swell. The more you push, the more they swell, until, like a balloon that has been blown up one time too many, they no longer collapse back to their normal size.

Sitting on a toilet for too long also gives you hemorrhoids. The longer you sit with your anus suspended over that grand canyon of your toilet, the more gravity pulls at the veins there and they swell. So sit down, do what you have to do, and get up. The bathroom is not the place to read *War and Peace*. If it is the only spot where you can be left alone to read, then put a chair in a closet, hang a good light there, and lock the door. You may be back in the closet, but at least you're less likely to get hemorrhoids.

If you're sitting on the toilet unable to go, get up, walk around, and don't sit back down until you feel the urge again. Not only will walking help prevent hemorrhoids, it will also stimulate colonic motility and, with it, a bowel movement.

Internal hemorrhoids are not caused by anal sex, but it can certainly irritate them and cause bleeding. (Use your imagination.) If hemorrhoids are a problem and you want to have anal sex, choose a water-soluble lubricant, make sure your partner is gentle, and try lying on your stomach, a position that will decrease vein swelling.

Hemorrhoids can certainly make you miserable, but if you follow a few simple steps, you probably can avoid surgery. First and foremost, keep your bowel movements soft but formed. Diarrhea can be more irritating than a hard stool. I usually advise patients to try to achieve one soft bowel movement a day. Of course, this is not always appropriate for everyone. Some people naturally go every other or every third day. What is normal for your body is fine, as long as your stool is not hard when it finally passes. The opposite is also true. Some men (especially those on protease inhibitors) have more than one bowel movement a day. That is fine, too, as long as their stool is soft and *formed*.

To achieve one soft bowel movement a day, I advise patients to take stool lubricants and bulk agents. The most common stool softener is docusate sodium (Colace), a gelcap containing an oil that is not absorbed into your system. (So don't fret about extra pounds.) The oil stays in your digestive tract mixing with your stool so that it slips out easier. This decreases trauma to your hemorrhoids and promotes healing.

Plant fiber is an important, although often missing, part of our diet and is crucial in the treatment of most anorectal disorders. The fiber is not absorbed into your system. Instead, it remains in your intestine, where it absorbs water and holds it in your stool. Your stool is bulkier, softer, and less traumatic as it passes over inflamed hemorrhoids. Fiber also shortens the transit time of feces through your colon and has been shown to decrease colon cancer rates.

I'm sure you've heard some elderly person expound on the virtues of prunes in producing "regularity." This is because prunes contain a lot of fiber. Other foods similarly high in fiber include vegetables, fruits, and unprocessed grains. Lettuce, contrary to popular belief, contains very little fiber. (But spinach and cabbage do.)

Because the typical "American" diet is long on junk food and short on fiber, I advise taking bulk agents that are natural fiber supplements. Psyllium husk, the most common fiber supplement, is available in health food stores as well as in commercial preparations. Metamucil, Fibercon, and Citrucel are common brands available in powder, wafer, or tablet form. They contain varying amounts of fiber with sugar or nonsugar sweeteners, so read labels carefully (especially if you don't want sugar) and choose the preparation that works best for you. Start with a single evening dose, because initially fiber supplements promote gas. Once you can tolerate a daily dose, increase it to twice a day. Fiber supplements are not habit-forming laxatives. Drink plenty of liquid when taking a fiber supplement. As mentioned, the fiber absorbs water and holds it in your stool. If you just take fiber and don't drink enough water, the fiber remains dry; the end result is something akin to shitting the proverbial brick.

Not only is it important that your stool be of the right consistency, it must not contain any irritants. Most of us are unaware of how caustic stools can be to our sensitive anorectal tissues. People with hemorrhoids often know that certain foods bring on an attack. If you know what bothers you, eliminate it from your diet. (See "Anal Pruritus (Itch)" for a list of common food offenders.)

When hemorrhoids flare, topical creams and ointments often provide relief. Preparation H and other common over-the-counter medications may help soothe swollen tissue. Choose a cream containing 1 to 1.5 percent hydrocortisone, which doesn't require a prescription. If you want a stronger and often more effective 2.5 percent hydrocortisone cream, you will need to consult your physician for a prescription.

I am often asked which is more effective, a suppository or cream. Obviously for an external problem, use a cream applied directly to your irritated area. If your main complaint is bleeding hemorrhoids, then a suppository or cream with an applicator for insertion into your rectum is most effective. Start with a suppository at bedtime, but if your symptoms are severe, morning-and-evening dosing may be necessary.

I have also found that medicated pads such as Tucks can help reduce swelling and soothe irritation. If pain and swelling are severe, you may get added relief if you keep pads in the refrigerator and apply them cold directly to your anus.

The sitz bath is another mainstay of hemorrhoid treatment. It involves submerging your anal area in warm water—bath temperature, not scalding. (Remember, we are not making chicken soup here.) The warm water helps reduce swelling and relaxes your anal sphincter, which can go into spasm during hemorrhoid flare-ups. Fancy and often expensive sitz bath attachments that hook up to the toilet are available in most pharmacies and surgical supply stores. You don't need a prescription to buy them, but a simple bathtub is just as effective and may also relax your whole body in the process.

Men with particularly painful hemorrhoid attacks often constipate themselves to prevent the pain a trip to the bathroom brings. This is one of the worst things to do. When your bowel movement finally does come—as it must—it will be as hard as a rock and more damaging to your already inflamed anus.

One patient I treated discovered that constipation was definitely not the way to go when his hemorrhoids flared and tried laxatives instead. Also not a good idea. He called screaming after his first episode of diarrhea because his ass felt like it was on fire. Laxatives are highly caustic. When passed with diarrhea, they burn your already inflamed hemorrhoids.

If hemorrhoids do not resolve within a few days, then consult a doctor. Your physician may recommend a number of possible treatments, so know your options.

Surgical removal is the only option for external hemorrhoids. Since they have pain receptors, they cannot be burned or rubber-banded or treated by any of the other modalities commonly used for internal hemorrhoids. Many physicians will tell you that your hemorrhoids do not need to be treated—particularly if you are dealing with anal tags (from a prior thrombosed external hemorrhoid or chronic irritation). This is good advice. When a hemorrhoid is removed surgically, the area becomes inflamed from bacteria that pass in the stool. This inflammation can leave you with another tag in place of the one your doctor removed. I tell patients that their anus will never be as smooth as the day they were born, because it just doesn't heal that way. As long as you understand this, you can make a sound decision.

Internal hemorrhoids don't sense pain, so treatment options differ. The following are the most common treatments physicians recommend and usually are performed right in their offices:

❖ Rubber-band ligation. A rubber band is shot around the hemorrhoid through a small instrument inserted into your anus. Although generally painless, the hemorrhoid dies because the rubber band stops blood flow to it. (The hemorrhoid is essentially strangled.) You may notice a little bleeding and discomfort. Usually only one hemorrhoid is treated at a time, so multiple trips to the doctor are required.

◇ Infrared photocoagulation or cautery. Both treatments involve the same principle: The blood supply to the hemorrhoid is clotted off (either by infrared light or electricity) and it dies. Again, discomfort is usually minimal (you may feel some heat), and multiple trips to the doctor are required. Beware of doctors who tell you that infrared photocoagulation is the same as laser surgery—it is not.

◇ Sclerotherapy. This treatment is especially common for internal hemorrhoids among older physicians, whereby a caustic fluid is injected into each hemorrhoid and causes the blood to clot (sclerose). Hemorrhoids die and eventually slough. Most physicians tackle only one hemorrhoid at a time.

None of these three treatments will rid you of your external hemorrhoids, all require multiple visits to your doctor over several weeks, and all are not as effective for long-term eradication as a standard surgical hemorrhoidectomy, whereby your entire hemorrhoid is cut away. On the plus side, however, these procedures are less painful with quicker recovery than standard surgical techniques and can be performed right in the doctor's office. You probably won't even miss a day of work. Your external hemorrhoids (if any) can be removed with local anesthesia once your internal hemorrhoids are gone.

Surgical removal, whether performed with a knife or laser, is the most effective and permanent way to eliminate hemorrhoids. It is also the most painful. I had a patient who would rather stand on his head after every bowel movement until his hemorrhoids went back inside his anus than have surgery. He finally consented to surgery when he developed a back problem from his contortions. Invariably after surgery most patients tell me, "The first week was hell, but now that it's over I shouldn't have waited so long."

Although surgeons have made great strides in pain control and a hospital stay is no longer required after a complete hemorrhoidectomy, do not expect to be up dancing for days. Surgery is usually reserved for the most severe cases where there is bleeding, an extensive external component, and/or hemorrhoids prolapse (hang) out of the anus.

A controversy rages among surgeons as to the efficacy of the laser over the knife. Lasers cause less damage and scarring to the anus. They seal small blood vessels and nerve endings, and some people report less pain after laser surgery. In the end what probably is more important is that you choose a skilled surgeon whom you can trust, whatever his surgical method.

A beefy patient lay across my examining table insisting that I remove his external hemorrhoid. I squinted and moved from side to side, trying to imagine how this barely visible nubbin of extra skin could possibly be causing him any problems. "It's so tiny," I said. "There's no reason to remove it."

"I want it off. It shows up in my close-ups."

Because for many gay men, their anus and rectum function as sexual organs, this fact may affect what constitutes optimal treatment for hemorrhoids. Some men complain that even the smallest hemorrhoid impairs their sex life and they want it removed. It is important to talk to your doctor about this and ask for guidelines about resuming anal sex after treatment. Porno stars aside, it is important that you realize that anal tags and mild hemorrhoids very often have no effect on anal intercourse (from a functional, not aesthetic, perspective), and it may be best to leave them alone.

Last, once you have had anal surgery, some scarring is

unavoidable and can cause tightening. Usually this is not a problem, and anal sex can resume with a gentle touch without difficulty after healing occurs (four to eight weeks after a standard hemorrhoidectomy). Occasionally patients who undergo surgery for extensive hemorrhoids will need rectal dilators to stretch their opening to once again accommodate their partner. (See Chapter 1.) Even if you choose an in-office, nonsurgical method for removing internal hemorrhoids, you still will not be able to have anal sex until the area heals. This generally occurs within two weeks—unless you require additional treatments to remove multiple hemorrhoids.

Anal Fissure

An anal fissure is a tear or cut in the anal lining and usually begins as an extremely painful event. Most men with fissures complain of severe pain during bowel movements and a bright-red streak of blood on their stool. Pain can persist for hours after each bowel movement and results from spasm in the anal sphincter. (See Figure 2.1.) Anal fissures most often result from a hard bowel movement tearing the sensitive lining of the anal canal. Pain and bleeding often are incorrectly attributed to hemorrhoids, which, unless thrombosed, are rarely painful. In gay men, other common causes of fissures are trauma from anal intercourse or fingers and toys as well as ulcers related to HIV. Fissures usually occur in the posterior midline (the side of the anus closest to the coccyx, or tailbone), but if caused by sexual trauma, they can occur anywhere.

When fissures first occur, they look like a small cut at the anal opening and may be covered by a speck of blood. If untreated, stool rubbing over the cut deepens it and further intensifies the muscle spasm. Anal sphincter spasm tightens the anal opening, making it even harder to push out a bowel movement. The tear deepens, taking on the appearance of a tiny volcanic crater with white edges of callused skin. The cut can extend right down to the sphincter muscles. Often just the simple effort of spreading your cheeks apart for a close look can be painful. When fissures become chronic, the long-standing inflammation can cause a small anal tag (a sentinel pile) to form at your anal opening. (See Figure 2.1.) Many men incorrectly attribute their pain and bleeding to the tag, which is the result of the inflammation, not the cause. Usually the fissure can be seen just inside the anal opening. As with thrombosed hemorrhoids, constipating yourself or using laxatives only makes the problem worse.

A patient walked into my office demanding surgery for his anal fissure. He insisted that it still hurt like hell despite stool softeners. When I questioned him, I discovered he had been taking glasses of milk to keep his bowels soft instead of the medications I had advised. Obviously he suffered from lactose intolerance and was not digesting milk. His colonic bacteria worked on the undigested milk sugars, creating acid. The acid acted like a laxative and burned severely when it passed across his raw fissure. His fissure healed as soon as he switched to psyllium husk.

As in the treatment of hemorrhoids, initial treatment of an acute fissure is conservative (nonsurgical) and aimed at softening the stool and relaxing sphincter muscles. Because every hard bowel movement feels like a rock rubbing against your cut, use over-the-counter bulk agents containing psyllium husk and a stool softener like docusate sodium (Colace). When I tell patients with fissures that they need to have a bulkier stool, they usually look at me in wide-eyed terror. If it already hurts to move your bowels, why would you want a larger stool? Although initially painful, a soft, bulky stool conforms to the narrowed size of your anal opening and is less damaging to your healing cut. More than half the patients with acute anal fissures heal within several days after instituting appropriate treatment.

Over-the-counter creams, especially those with a steroid component, also may help heal fissures. Avoid suppositories, because inserting them across your cut through a tight sphincter exacerbates pain. When you push in the suppository you actually push it above your sphincter and fissure, past the point where it will do any good. Since fissures are most often right at your anal opening, creams can be applied directly with your fingertip or an applicator. Many creams include a topical anesthetic that will relieve pain and relax your sphincter.

Pain that is caused by a fissure is not only from the tear but also from muscle spasm. Therefore, in addition to softening your stool, it is important to relax your sphincter as much as possible. Obviously, the larger the anal opening, the easier it will be for your stool to pass. Warm sitz baths act directly on the area and help loosen muscles. If your spasm is severe, a muscle relaxant like Valium (diazepam) may help, and don't be afraid to ask your doctor for it. I do not recommend narcotic pain medications, which are constipating, but prefer topical anesthetics applied directly to the fissure. In addition to deadening pain, they also relax sphincters.

If a fissure occurs during anal sex, stop immediately. Avoid any attempt at further intercourse or manipulation of the anus until healing occurs. If pain is severe or if fever develops, it could mean that a penis (or toy) tore through your sphincter into the delicate tissue surrounding your anus. Seek medical attention immediately, because infection will usually result and antibiotics and/or surgery will be required.

A chronic fissure is less likely than an acute fissure to heal on its own. Recent medical studies show that topical nitrates applied to the cut promote healing. Many people with heart disease use nitrates applied in patches to their skin to keep their coronary arteries open. With fissures, nitrates are thought to dilate blood vessels in the area, bringing in more nutrients and oxygen to promote healing. In doses used for heart disease, nitrates cause severe headaches and other troubling side effects. Unfortunately, the medication is not yet commercially available in reduced strength, so consult your physician.

Some surgeons promote healing by cauterizing fissures. Although you may wince at the painful sound of the word, cauterization is performed in your doctor's office with only a topical anesthetic. The doctor uses a weak electric current or chemical to burn the area. Expect to need several treatments over a four- to eight-week period. Results have been spotty at best.

The sphincterotomy is the mainstay of surgical treatment for anal fissures. When a fissure becomes chronic, your sphincter muscle, through its spasms, has been in a perpetual workout and is much stronger than it needs to be. This added strength tightens your anus to the point where any bowel movement is traumatic and the fissure will never heal. A sphincterotomy cuts a portion of the muscle to weaken it, breaking the spasm and widening your opening.

To better understand the process, try thinking of the anal sphincter as your biceps muscle. (Just try!) Before you start weight training, you can press only sixty pounds. With exercise, your muscle mass increases so that you can lift double the weight. If a surgeon removed a piece of your biceps, you might be able to lift only sixty pounds once again. This is exactly what a sphincterotomy accomplishes.

The surgery is performed on an outpatient basis (you go home right after it) and requires only a local anesthetic. Don't be frightened, though. Most surgeons combine local anesthesia with intravenous drugs that relax you and make you drowsy. You'll be high as a kite and not remember anything.

Once you are on the operating table, your internal sphincter muscle is relaxed by cutting away a small portion at its very end. Most muscle above the fissure is left intact, as is the external sphincter. You're probably concerned that incontinence (inability to control your bowels) will result, and rightfully so. That is indeed one of the risks of the surgery. You must rely on the skill of your surgeon to cut just enough muscle to break your spasm without causing incontinence. Thankfully, incontinence is rare because so little muscle is actually cut. If you do have trouble, usually it is only with controlling flatus (gas) immediately after surgery, and that improves with time. (Approximately one-third of patients who have had a sphincterotomy complain of incontinence of flatus immediately after surgery. This drops to less than 5 percent by the second week. The rate of fecal incontinence is even lower.) As with any surgery, choose your surgeon carefully.

After any anorectal surgery, many patients report incontinence when the problem really is their inability to hold back a bowel movement because of soreness. Your rectum stores stool until it is convenient for you to eliminate it. After surgery your sphincter works well, but when a piece of stool touches the fresh cut, your muscles relax to get out of the way. You perceive this sudden urge to move your bowels as incontinence, when really it is more like you're pulling a cut hand away from a rock.

In rare instances, you might find a surgeon who recommends a simple anal dilatation, or "stretch," to treat your fissure. Although this procedure is more popular in the United Kingdom, some surgeons in this country prefer it to a sphincterotomy. In essence, the surgeon stretches your tight sphincter until it partially tears. Most surgeons frown on this method because tearing occurs in an uncontrolled manner. With a sphincterotomy, the surgeon knows exactly how much muscle is cut. In theory, an anal dilatation should result in a higher incidence of postoperative incontinence, but that hasn't been shown to be the case. If a surgeon recommends an anal dilatation, it may be that in *his* hands this is the best way to treat your problem. Surgeons are best at doing the type of surgery they have experience in.

Gay men who practice anoreceptive intercourse may develop an acute fissure from direct injury. If treated with stool softeners and abstinence, this type of fissure should heal. If, however, a chronic fissure develops and surgery is required, then a sphincterotomy or anal dilatation is usually not necessary. Most often men who have had anal intercourse have already stretched their sphincter (I'm sure you can figure out how) and spasm is rarely present. The fissure usually will heal if the surgeon removes the scar tissue and closes the tear with a few stitches. Keep this in mind if a surgeon tells you a sphincterotomy is necessary. In this instance, you might be placing yourself at a higher risk for incontinence because your sphincter is already loose. You can always go back for a sphincterotomy if your fissure doesn't heal after simple closure.

HIV-positive patients often present with many different types of anal fissures that are atypical and quite complicated. HIV and medications used to treat it may cause diarrhea and subsequent fissure formation. The constant wet stool macerates the anal lining and promotes breakdown and tearing. (Think of your mushy skin after you've soaked in a tub for too long.) Bulk agents and medications that control diarrhea (Imodium) often will cure this type of fissure.

Although many times rectal bleeding and pain are the hallmark symptoms of HIV-related fissures, you may notice only a chronic purulent (infected) discharge and foul odor.

Your discharge may appear as a brownish-green stain in your underwear. This type of HIV-related fissure looks different from typical anal fissures and more closely resembles a broad, shallow ulcer rather than a simple cut. As with any new symptom, if you have pain and an infected discharge, tell your physician.

If you have HIV and a fissure, first treat it with topical steroid creams, stool softeners, and bulk agents. If healing does not occur, as is often the case, then the ulcer may need to be biopsied and removed. In these instances, your ulcer may result from many different HIV-related causes, including the HIV virus itself, tuberculosis, CMV, herpes, fungus infection, syphilis, lymphoma, Kaposi's sarcoma, or other cancers.

I saw a young HIV-positive man whose fissures had been treated with creams and suppositories for two years by another doctor. He gripped the table prepared for pain as I slid my finger into his anus.

I apologized for hurting him, but he said, "It'll be worth it if you can just help me."

My heart sank. I felt his fissure, and I also felt the cancer that caused it.

As a gay man with HIV, you may find yourself faced with a chronic, debilitating anal ulcer and a surgeon who refuses to operate on you. Oftentimes the medical community cites poor healing in HIV-positive patients as a reason for not treating their ulcers. Although this may be the case, if your immune status is relatively good, you should heal after surgery. Whenever faced with a physician who says "Sorry, but you'll have to live with it," get another opinion. You'll probably find someone who'll help you. I caution you, however, not to be too optimistic. Many times, even though your ulcer is removed and studied under a microscope, no cause for it is ever identified. However, simple removal may be enough to cure it. Of course, if something treatable turns up (such as a tumor or virus), you will no doubt require further therapy.

Abscess and Fistula-in-Ano

An abscess in your anal region is potentially very dangerous, yet often gay men ignore it until it progresses to a critical stage. An abscess begins as a painful sensation in your anal area, which gay men often wrongly attribute to a prior sexual experience. Embarrassment keeps them from seeing a physician while their infection is still in its early stages. Although the infection certainly could be caused by injury during sex, most often it results from a piece of stool getting caught in your anal crypts (glands). (See Figure 2.1.) This earliest painful stage is called a *cryptitis*. As infection progresses, it can spread into sphincter muscles and fatty tissue around the anus and rectum. The infection forms a cavity and pus accumulates. At this point you have what is commonly called a perirectal abscess.

Once an abscess develops, it burrows toward the skin, slowly destroying more and more tissue. Your skin reddens, is warm to the touch, and may feel like a water balloon if you gently push on it. Of course, any pressure to the area is very painful. If a doctor does not intervene, eventually your abscess will break through the skin and pus will pour out. Although you'll feel better immediately, your problem won't be solved, because the hole is not large enough to drain the cavity fully. Pus reaccumulates until it drains again, but the unabated infection destroys more and more surrounding tissue, including, occasionally, the sphincters. I have treated patients whose infection left them unable to control their bowels.

Proper treatment for a perirectal abscess is surgical and is called an I&D (incision and drainage). While antibiotics often are necessary, by themselves they are not enough. Local anesthesia for surgery won't provide adequate relief. Ask to either go to sleep (general anesthesia) or have regional anesthesia that numbs your lower body. Most people feel much better after their surgery.

I treated a young man who noticed severe rectal pressure several days after anal sex. He assumed that his problem was related to something that happened during sex and put off seeing a physician until he had a high fever and could barely walk. In his case, the abscess had traveled upward along his colon rather than out toward his skin. His abscess required multiple surgeries over more than two years until it was completely cured.

A fistula-in-ano can result from a prior abscess but is more often caused by a milder infection that never formed a full-blown cavity. Instead, the infection burrowed to your skin and popped open like a pimple. (See Figure 2.1.) Again, it is *rarely* related to a previous sexual experience. Most men complain of a tiny painful pimple or boil beside their anal opening that swells until it drains a bit of pus. Symptoms are rarely severe enough to see a doctor and may go away for days to months at a time until the cycle begins again.

A fistula-in-ano should be treated. If it blocks up and cannot drain, an abscess will develop. Some men have fistulas that form side tracks that spread around their anus making multiple holes (commonly called a watering-can anus). I have seen men with holes so large that stool came out of them when they moved their bowels. Not a pretty sight.

Surgery is the best treatment and involves opening the fistula (performing a fistulotomy) and removing debris so it can heal from the inside out. Usually discomfort after surgery is minimal. If the fistula is large and travels through sphincter muscles, incontinence is possible after surgery. In these cases, the surgery is much more complicated and done in stages. Occasionally, if faced with a very difficult fistula, a surgeon might recommend that it be left alone. Fortunately these extreme conditions are rare.

Anal Pruritus (Itch)

Advertisements for hemorrhoid remedies teach us that hemorrhoids itch. In fact, however, hemorrhoids often are the *result* of the itch, not the cause. Sure, huge internal hemorrhoids that hang out of your anus secreting mucus will itch. But these cases are rare. Most often chronic irritation causes the external tags you feel at your anal opening when you scratch. If a surgeon performs a hemorrhoidectomy, the tags may be gone temporarily, but your itch will remain. You continue to scratch and tags blossom once again.

Anal pruritis (itch) most often results from chronic skin irritation. Although the itch may be from psoriasis or an infection (see Chapters 3 and 4), a contact or allergic dermatitis is the most frequent cause. In other words, something your anal skin contacts irritates the hell out of it. Contact can come in the form of creams or perfumes applied before sex, scented or harsh soaps used for bathing or laundry, or an irritating food product coming out in your stool. When I mention this, most patients say, "It's never given me any problem before, so why should it now?" Most often something your body tolerated in the past has suddenly sensitized your skin and an allergy results.

With anal pruritis, the skin around the anus appears reddened and cracked. Over time, the skin thickens and takes on a more callused appearance. The itch worsens at night, and often cuts and scabs appear from scratching during sleep.

While steroid creams (prescription strength) will stop the

itch, long-term use weakens the skin. Suppositories have little effect since they travel up too far and bypass the problem. Instead, determine what caused your itch and eliminate it. The following are a few steps that can go a long way in resolving your problem. While some of them are quite difficult, if you can follow these procedures for just one month, you'll be well on your way to solving the problem.

- ❖ Eliminate any oils, creams, lotions, lubricants, and caustic soaps that come in contact with your anal region. This means changing your bath and laundry detergents. (If you use a laundry service, check to see what they wash your clothes in.)
- ❖ Don't use toilet paper. Toilet tissues contain bleaches and perfumes that can irritate skin. Try using Tucks, which are perfume-free pads containing witch hazel and can be purchased in most drugstores and supermarkets. In addition to removing fecal residue, they soothe the skin. Do not use the baby-wipe–type pads, as many contain irritating perfumes and alcohol.
- ❖ After you thoroughly cleanse the area, apply a thin layer of Balneol lotion. It soothes and lubricates the skin. If you sweat a lot, place a small piece of fluffed-up cotton against your anal opening to absorb moisture.
- ❖ Wipe with Tucks and apply Balneol in the morning when you awaken, just before bed, and after every bowel movement. And yes, you will have to take the wipes and lotion to work if that is where you have a bowel movement.
- ❖ Now comes the hard part. Eliminate all foods that can irritate your skin when they come out in your stool. The following is a list of the most common offenders:

    1. Acidic foods and their juices (tomato, orange, grapefruit, and other citrus fruits, etc.)
    2. Spicy foods (hot pepper, garlic, etc.)

3. Alcohol (Sorry, boys, no drinking—especially wine.)
4. Caffeine (Don't forget, tea, chocolate, and colas contain caffeine.)
5. Milk products (If you don't digest them well, bacteria in your colon convert the lactose to acid.) Yogurt with natural cultures and lactose-free milk are fine.

Try this for a month and I am willing to bet that your itch disappears completely or at least becomes tolerable. Once you reach this stage, begin to add back foods to your diet in the order that you miss them, one at a time. In other words, if you can't live without your morning coffee, then start with that. If after a week you are still not itching, then add something else. If your itch returns, then you can bet that you've discovered the culprit. Eliminating it from your diet may leave you itch free without using messy creams.

Occasionally the itch doesn't go away. Please remember that I have cited only the most common irritants. What bothers *your* skin might be unique. I remember a young man bursting into tears when I recited my standard list of foods to avoid. No, he wasn't a drama queen, but he had tried everything to no avail and couldn't take it anymore. He even slept in gloves to keep from tearing his skin apart in his sleep. Through careful discussion, I learned that he took many vitamins each day. When he cut them out (vitamin C is the most irritating), his itch disappeared. Artificial sweeteners caused the itch in another patient. Examine your diet and eliminate anything you eat in great amounts.

And what if the itch still doesn't go away? See your doctor, because something more serious might be going on. A parasite or something requiring a biopsy and prescription medication could be causing your problem.

Fecal Soiling

Most of us know the embarrassment of finding brown stains in our underwear or the "skid marks" of our youth. Often it occurs because we do not or cannot clean our anal area well enough to remove all fecal residue. For some, it is a time issue—it takes too long to get everything off, especially when confronted with bothersome external hemorrhoids. Just as wiping too long and too hard can damage sensitive anal skin, so too can not wiping enough. Fecal waste, whether solid or loose, can be very caustic. The itching or burning that results can become so severe that it interferes with your life.

When fecal soiling results from your inability to clean yourself properly, abandon toilet paper and use a wet tissue or cotton ball instead. They are far less abrasive and better at removing solid waste. Tucks are also effective and quite soothing. Do not use oil-based or perfumed products, which can be more irritating. Oils occlude pores and increase your chance of infection.

For some men, fecal soiling occurs throughout the day—especially when they pass gas. Sometimes they actually feel liquid or mucus seep out; other times they just see a brownish stain on their underwear. Some seepage is normal after receptive anal sex because your sphincter muscle is stretched and cannot contract, and also because fucking stimulates colonic motility, which sends feces from your colon down into your lower rectum. If you use an enema before anal sex and are bothered by seepage afterward, stop the enemas. An enema puts liquid into your rectum, and it is not entirely expelled before sex.

Some men have soiling even without anal sex or diarrhea. Treatment goals include keeping their anal area dry and eliminating waste from the rectum. After each bowel movement, wipe with a moist pad to remove any remaining residue. If you suffer from diarrhea, oral medications that constipate help. I also advise a consultation with a nutritionist to eliminate foods that promote loose stool and gas. Many times the simple act of expelling gas forces out mucus or liquid stool with it.

A diaper is rarely necessary, but you may get relief by placing a menstrual-type pad in the back of your underwear. The pad absorbs moisture and waste and helps keep you dry. When a patient looks at me in disbelief over the prospect of buying feminine hygiene pads, I tell him to butch it up and pretend he is the concerned spouse shopping for his wife. (So what if your wife's name is Tom?)

In heavier men with a fuller "caboose," so to speak, pads may not reach their anal opening well enough to keep them dry. In these individuals, a pad plus a fluffed-up cotton ball placed directly against their opening helps absorb moisture throughout the day. A mild steroid cream or Balneol may be needed, at least initially, if skin irritation is severe.

If soiling persists, I suggest a course of rectal wash-outs to remove residual feces after bowel movements. Particularly in patients with solid stools, seepage can occur because a bowel movement ends too soon, leaving waste in the rectum that leaks out at inopportune moments. The treatment? Insert an ear syringe filled with warm water and coated with a water-soluble lubricant into your rectum. (See Chapter 1.) Squeeze it gently several times to wash out any residual feces from your anal canal. Try this after each bowel movement for several days, then wait to see if your problem has resolved. Frequent irrigations are rarely necessary and do not have the same detrimental effect on your colon as full enemas do.

Profuse sweating in hot weather or after strenuous exercise loosens fecal residue present on your perianal skin and can be confused with fecal seepage. In this instance, your problem is not caused by seepage but by improper cleansing. For relief, wipe well before exercise and use a fluffed-up cotton ball to absorb sweat.

Fungal Dermatitis

Although fungal dermatitis is infectious, it is not sexually transmitted, so I am including it in this section. Two types of fungus infections typically involve your anogenital region. Tinea cruris, or jock itch as it is commonly called, typically occurs in sweat-prone areas with deep skin folds. Your anus and groin are prime targets, and you'll notice reddened skin and severe itch. Over-the-counter preparations such as Cruex and Lotrimin, to name just a few, are a good treatment for jock itch. I find that creams work better than sprays or powders for active infections.

Candida infections are also common in the anogenital region, particularly in men with HIV and diabetes. Those prone to chronic soiling or needing sitz baths who do not dry themselves properly afterward are also at risk. Redness and burning are the principal symptoms of fungal infection caused by *Candida albicans*. Skin is raw, and the infection acquires a well-demarcated red line at its outer border. It is important to differentiate a candida infection from jock itch, because treatment is different. Prescription antifungal creams such as nystatin or miconazole cure candida infections.

Bacterial Dermatitis

Bacterial dermatitis is a nonsexually transmitted infection. It occurs particularly after shaving, scratching, or rubbing your anogenital area and involves infection of the skin, hair follicles, and/or glands with streptococcus and staphylococcus bacteria. After shaving, nicks and follicles become infected and tiny pustules appear. Prescription antibiotics are required (oral or topical), and you must stop shaving until it heals.

Summary

At some point in your life you probably will develop a problem in your anus or rectum. Straight men as well as gay men suffer from anorectal disorders, and embarrassment should not prevent you from seeking medical attention. Most of the time anal sex did *not* cause your problem.

- ⬥ Rectal bleeding that persists for more than three days or returns should be evaluated by a physician.
- ⬥ Stool softeners and bulk agents combined with steroid creams or suppositories will cure most anorectal disorders. Surgery is rarely necessary.
- ⬥ Fever or severe pain requiring analgesic medication (even aspirin or acetaminophen) is a serious symptom. See a physician immediately.
- ⬥ Ignoring a problem increases your risk that surgery will be needed.
- ⬥ If you are HIV positive and a surgeon tells you that there is nothing to be done, get another opinion.
- ⬥ If surgery is considered, be sure to discuss all options with your doctor so you can determine which procedure is best for you.
- ⬥ If you've had anal sex, tell your doctor. If you can't, then find a doctor you can be honest with.

CHAPTER 3

Nonviral Sexually Transmitted Diseases—

OR BUGS AND BACTERIA,

THE TWO B'S

He zipped up his pants, his expression clearly troubled. "I don't know how I got this," he said. "I mean, my sex is so safe it's practically nonexistent."

I smiled. "Nevertheless, you've got a discharge and I bet it's gonorrhea. We won't know for sure until the culture comes back, but it's best to treat you anyway." I cleared my throat. "There's something else. You've got to notify your sexual partners."

"That's just it, there aren't any. Not since Brian and I broke up."

I shook my head. "You didn't get this from a toilet seat. You must have slept with someone."

"No . . . well, I did get a blow job from this guy. That can't give it to you, can it?"

We all know how prevalent sexually transmitted diseases are among men who have sex with men; now we need to learn how to prevent them. But first, we must have a thorough understanding of each disease, its route of transmission, and its signs and symptoms. Nonviral STDs are still the most common, but in the last decade, they have certainly been overshadowed by AIDS. The pity is that these diseases are virtually 100 percent curable, but without treatment they can be lethal. Unfortunately, as our focus has shifted to AIDS, both physicians and gay men are less aware of these problems. In effect, what we are now seeing is our failure to treat curable infections because physicians and patients don't know about them. And don't think for a minute that syphilis and gonorrhea are no longer a threat. They're out there in daunting numbers, and the longer it takes to make the correct diagnosis, the greater the chance infection will spread between unaware partners. As we saw with HIV, transmission is exponential.

Syphilis

Why, you ask, am I bothering to mention a historic disease, virtually extinct in our very modern times? Because syphilis is far from gone. An estimated 101,000 new cases were reported last year in this country, and half were thought to be in men who have sex with men. That's more than the yearly estimated new cases of HIV. According to the Centers for Disease Control in Atlanta, Baltimore had the dubious distinction of having the most cases of syphilis for 1997 in this country. (Anyone thinking of moving?)

Although legend has it that syphilis was carried to Europe from the Western Hemisphere by Columbus's crew, this probably was not the case. Descriptions of venereal diseases with characteristics similar to syphilis appear in ancient literature, and anthropologists have found signs of bone destruction in human prehistoric remains similar to what we see in late syphilis. Syphilis is caused by a spirochete type of bacteria called *Treponema pallidum.* It was first identified in 1905 by Fritz Schaudinn. The following year Dr. August von Wassermann developed a famous test for syphilis that bears his name and is still used today. The real breakthrough in syphilis treatment came in 1943, when penicillin first was used to treat the disease successfully.

Syphilis is transmitted through direct sexual contact between mucous membranes and, rarely, by close skin-to-skin contact. The organism cannot survive drying and is easily killed by soap and water. Infection most often occurs on the penis or anal canal after unprotected sex, but the mouth also can be a site. The first sign of syphilis is a *painless* red ulcer called a chancre at the site where the organism invaded the body. (See Figure 3.1.) On your penis, look for a chancre on or close to your glans (head), although it also can be on the shaft or scrotum. Chancres are extremely contagious. If you see one on your partner's penis, avoid sexual contact until he's treated. Unfortunately, it is nearly impossible to see a chancre within the anal canal without medical equipment.

Though usually single, chancres can be multiple and appear within ninety days after infection (average two to four weeks). At this stage, syphilis is diagnosed by collecting some clear fluid the ulcer weeps and examining it under a

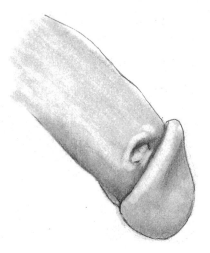

Figure 3.1: Syphilis Chancre

special darkfield microscope. This fluid teems with wiggling spirochetes. Unfortunately, most physicians don't own darkfield microscopes, since these days syphilis occurs relatively infrequently. Chancres heal by themselves without any treatment within three to eight weeks.

When syphilis infects the anus, the chancre may be painful and often misdiagnosed as a fissure. Anal syphilis frequently causes bloody bowel movements, diarrhea, and a mucus discharge. Many gay men undergo needless anal surgery (sometimes involving radical resections for a presumed cancer) because their doctors did not make the correct diagnosis—a frightening fact considering that the disease could have been cured with antibiotics alone.

Although a penile chancre has a fairly distinct appearance, it can be confused with other more common problems, such as genital herpes. A culture for the herpes virus provides an answer within a day or two, and if negative, think of syphilis. A penile or anal ulcer also can result from injury, but you or your partner usually will remember this.

After the chancre heals, syphilis enters a secondary stage as spirochetes spread throughout the body. Symptoms are similar to those of a viral illness: fever, joint pains, runny nose, and lethargy. Although copper-colored skin lesions can cover the body, they typically appear only on palms and soles. As syphilis spreads to other parts of the body, lymph node enlargement (swollen glands), liver enlargement, and eye and nervous system problems are also common. You are still infectious, but the disease is easily diagnosed through various tests that detect antibodies in your blood to the organism. The most common test is the VDRL (venereal disease research laboratory). If your VDRL is positive, infection is confirmed by the more sensitive, though harder to perform, FTA-ABS (fluorescent treponemal antibody absorption) test.

In approximately 40 percent of untreated patients, infection progresses to tertiary syphilis within ten to twenty years. Although no longer contagious, it can attack your nervous system (causing blindness, deafness, and insanity), or heart and major arteries (resulting in heart valve damage, aneurysm of the aorta, and cardiac failure). At this stage syphilis can be lethal.

Antibiotics cure primary or secondary syphilis; the most common is penicillin, given in one high-dose injection. For men allergic to penicillin, erythromycin or doxycycline taken orally for two weeks is an acceptable alternative. When syphilis remains untreated for more than a year, penicillin injections weekly for three weeks or oral antibiotics for one month are necessary. Occasionally in men with HIV, the disease is harder to eradicate and may require higher doses and prolonged administration of antibiotics.

If you have syphilis, you must be checked for other STDs as well. Very often, where there is one STD, there is also another. So if your physician hasn't already checked you for HIV, gonorrhea, and other STDs, ask that it be done.

Taking your antibiotic is not enough; all sexual partners you placed at risk must be notified and tested. Syphilis has been virtually eliminated from Canada, Sweden, and other industrialized countries. This notable accomplishment occurred only through vigorous screening, treatment, and notification of sexual partners. With the gay community's cooperation, this country can move a step closer to eliminating this terrible disease.

Gonorrhea

How about these frightening tidbits: Worldwide, gonorrhea is the most common STD, and in the United States it is the most commonly reported communicable disease. The Centers for Disease Control counted almost 1 million new cases of gonorrhea in 1997, while some researchers estimated that the number of unreported cases was more than double that. Gonorrhea is caused by a tiny bacterium called *Neisseria gonorrhoeae,* which won't grow in anything less than optimal conditions. It needs a warm, moist environment with high levels of carbon dioxide. The bacterium is extremely susceptible to drying and rarely transmitted outside of sex. Although sharing dildos can be risky, fingers, toilets, and saunas are usually safe.

Gonorrhea can infect the mouth, throat, urethra (the tube in your penis that carries urine and semen), and anal canal. Your anus becomes infected after anoreceptive intercourse with a man who has gonococcal urethritis. While kissing is probably safe, fellating an infected partner is not. Your urethra can be infected through insertive anal intercourse (but it is easier to give than to receive) or direct contact with a man's infected penis.

Gonorrhea most commonly infects your urethra, with symptoms beginning within two to five days. Most men complain of pain when urinating (dysuria) and a purulent (infected) penile discharge. The amount of the highly infectious discharge can vary. Some men notice green or yellow fluid dripping from their penis, while others only have a stain on their underwear. When examining a potential partner for signs of gonorrhea, the typical discharge usually can be distinguished from pre-cum because that tends to be clear. (See Chapter 10.)

The anorectal canal is another frequent site of gonorrhea, but because the infection is often painless, it may persist undiagnosed. In the anal canal, gonorrhea produces a discharge that often is first mistaken for leaking stool. Some men report blood or mucus in their bowel movements and discomfort.

When gonorrhea infects your mouth and throat, the symptoms may be similar to those of a typical strep throat, with redness, pain on swallowing, and enlarged lymph nodes. Most men are unaware of the seriousness of their oral infection.

Doctors often diagnose gonorrhea from "typical" symptoms and then confirm it by culture. Although the bacteria have a unique appearance under a microscope, most physicians lack the appropriate equipment in their offices. Therefore, most doctors sample your discharge with a cotton swab and send it to a laboratory for culture. The cultures must be handled carefully and in accordance with strict protocols, since the bacteria require optimal conditions for growth. DNA probes are another useful tool in diagnosing gonorrhea.

With a penile infection, your discharge is obtained by milking your urethra and culturing fluid that collects at the tip. If your discharge is not readily apparent, a physician may need to pass a tiny cotton swab about one inch into your urethra. I assure you that this procedure is more painful psychologically than physically. Your mouth and anus are easier to culture, requiring only a swab rubbed inside to collect any bacteria.

Make your physician aware of the possibility of gonorrhea before he examines you, because your mouth and anus can look perfectly normal. If your doctor suspects gonorrhea in one place, every orifice must be cultured, because the incidence of asymptomatic infections occurring at multiple sites is great. In other words, if you have it in one hole, you probably have it in another. Approximately 20 percent of patients with urethral gonorrhea also have oral gonorrhea.

Penicillin was the mainstay of gonorrhea treatment, but the bacteria have become increasingly resistant. Currently ceftriaxone, a cephalosporin type of antibiotic, given in a single injection is the drug of choice. Another class of antibiotics called quinolones (ciprofloxacin) are also effective and taken orally. Recently, however, reports have begun to surface in the medical literature documenting a growing resistance to these antibiotics as well. Close monitoring will tell if quinolones remain effective in the future.

Failure to treat gonorrhea is dangerous, because you continue to transmit infection to unsuspecting partners, and the bacteria can spread throughout your body. Gonorrhea frequently targets the joints, skin, heart, and occasionally brain. You'll need higher doses of antibiotics over a longer period to cure these infections.

As with syphilis, your physician must check you for other STDs. Gonorrhea is frequently associated with HIV, anal warts, herpes, and other forms of urethritis. Disturbing evidence suggests that men with gonorrhea are at increased risk for catching and transmitting HIV. Gonorrhea probably makes it easier for HIV to pass through inflamed mucous membranes into your blood. As with all STDs, you must notify any sexual partners you placed at risk so that they can be tested.

Pediculosis Pubis (the Crabs)

Pediculosis pubis (more commonly called the crabs) is caused by an infestation of pubic lice (*Phthirius pubis*). Lice are extremely contagious and easily passed between partners through close physical contact. (Rubbing is more than enough.) Even sharing a bed or towel with an infected man may be enough for you to catch lice. A condom certainly won't protect you no matter when you put it on. Knowing this, you can easily understand how infestation occurs with just seemingly harmless touching.

Infestation occurs when a louse (bug, not guy) comes in contact with your pubic or perianal hair. On hairier men, lice may spread to their upper thighs and lower abdomen. Occasionally they can even be found in axillary hair (armpits), beard, or mustache.

The louse bites at the base of hair follicles and feasts almost continuously on blood. Intense itching is the key symptom and results from the body's allergic response to the bites. If you have been infected before, your body is already sensitized and itching begins almost immediately. If, however, you are one of the lucky ones and this is your first experience as a louse cafeteria, then it may take up to a week before you begin to scratch. Bacterial skin infections develop from your scratching, not from the lice.

No microscope or fancy blood tests are needed to diagnose a lice infestation, only a look at your pubic area. It is rare to actually see a louse (a rust-colored speck on your skin), because most infestations contain fewer than twenty adult lice. Instead of actual bugs, look for dark-red specks of louse poop on your skin and underwear or nits (eggs) attached to your pubic hair. The eggs laid by the female are cemented to your hair at skin level. As the hair grows, the egg moves out with it. Eggs appear as small white or dark specks on your pubic hair. Although they can be mistaken for skin flakes or kinks in the hairs, the associated itching should give you a clue that something more serious is going on.

You can debug yourself at home with various over-the-counter medications. Nix, RID, and Kwell are some of the more common preparations available in shampoo or lotion form. Follow the directions on the box, being careful to shampoo or rub the lotion over all potential sites (pubic, scrotal, anal, and axillary hair), and leave it in place for the required time. Some physicians believe lotions are more effective than shampoos, while most men prefer to shampoo. Complete your treatment by running a fine "nit" comb through your pubic hair to remove any killed eggs. Most medications are strong enough to kill adult lice and eggs with one application, and a second treatment is necessary one week later *only* if eggs persist.

Some men worry their treatment failed because itching persists. This is a normal phenomenon, for the itch usually takes several days to disappear. Be patient and stay calm.

The towel you dry off with and the clothes you put on after treatment must be fresh or you risk reinfestation. Wash all your linens and clothes in hot water, then iron them or spin them in the dryer on high heat to kill any remaining lice.

As with any STD, you must notify any partners at risk for infection. Remember, only close contact is necessary (even if you just shared a towel), not intercourse. And last, it is easy for you to diagnose and treat crabs in the privacy of your home without seeing a physician. I urge you, however, to notify your doctor and get tested for other STDs, because at least one-third of men have a concurrent STD.

Scabies

Scabies are another sexually transmitted infestation. A small mite called *Sarcoptes scabiei* burrows into your skin, builds a nest, and raises a family. Not a pretty picture. Your hands, particularly the web spaces between your fingers, are common sites, and so are your genitals, arms, and abdomen. Intense itching that worsens at night is characteristic, and transmission occurs through direct contact or sharing a bed with an infected partner. The diagnosis is made either by seeing the burrows the parasite makes into your skin or by skin biopsy. Prescription creams such as lindane (Kwell) as well as a thorough washing of all linens and clothes kills the mite. Remember to notify any of your partners at risk for infection and get tested for other STDs.

Summary

Unfortunately, as our attention focuses on HIV, doctors and patients alike are less aware of the other highly prevalent yet curable infections. Men go untreated because their problem is not diagnosed.

◈ If you have one STD, get checked for others.

◈ Notify all partners at risk so they can be tested and, if necessary, treated.

◈ Even though a chancre will go away without treatment, you still have syphilis.

◈ Gonorrhea in your anus and mouth is much harder to diagnose than in your penis.

◈ Penetration or ejaculation is not required for the transmission of these infections—close sexual contact is enough.

◈ Don't forget to wash all clothes and linens in hot water after a case of crabs or scabies.

CHAPTER 4

Non-HIV Viral Sexually Transmitted Diseases—

OR HIV ISN'T THE ONLY

VIRUS OUT THERE!

I washed my hands and turned to face my patient.
"They're hemorrhoids, right, Doc?" he asked.
"No," I said. *"They're definitely not hemorrhoids. You've got venereal warts."*
He pointed to his index finger. "Could they be from my hands? I had a wart burned off there several months ago."
"No, you got these warts from sex."
"Impossible. I only have safe sex. Always a condom. You can't get it with a condom, can you?"

In the AIDS era, most guys are so worried about HIV that they forget about all the other viral sexually transmitted diseases. Although the list is long, the most common viral STDs include herpes, condyloma, and molluscum. (No, it's not something you'd order at a raw bar.) I have included hepatitis in this chapter because within the gay community, this disease is often spread through sexual contact. As we saw in Chapter 3, most STDs are far more prevalent than AIDS and don't require ejaculation or even penetration to spread. Viral STDs are no exception, but it gets worse; the condom you so faithfully wear for penetration may not protect you. If your partner has been rubbing his penis against your butt or groin, he can easily pass a virus. You say it couldn't happen because you make him wear a condom even during foreplay. Don't forget about his scrotum, pubic hair, and base of his shaft, areas not covered by the condom. He can carry viruses there and give them to you. And once you catch one of these nasty viruses, you can have it for life.

This doesn't mean you are doomed to a life of pain and unsightly blisters. On the contrary, viral STDs are typified by recurring outbreaks between quiet periods. These viruses hide within your cells, safe from marauding antibodies, white blood cells, and medications.

A virus is the simplest biological form—a segment of genetic material tightly wrapped inside a protein coat. Unable to reproduce on its own, a virus must invade a living cell to multiply. Once safe inside, the virus commandeers the cell's reproductive machinery and new viruses are made. When a virus is dormant in a cell, its genetic material is still present but idle until it receives some unknown biological stimulus to reproduce again. Then the cells are turned into factories making copies of the virus. New viruses break out of the cells (sometimes but not always destroying the cell in the process) and move to infect other cells—in your body or in an unsuspecting partner!

Each viral outbreak sends your immune system into overdrive, churning out antibodies and T-cells that attack viruses. Men with AIDS may not have immune systems capable of producing enough T-cells to kill the virus. Fortunately, various medications such as acyclovir (Zovirax) help immune systems by preventing viral reproduction and are available by prescription.

Since there is no simple way to rid yourself of many of the viral STDs, what's a sexually active gay man to do? The answer is simple: Prevent infection in the first place. But prevention is a two-sided responsibility. You must recognize signs of infection in your partner (see Chapter 10), and you also must recognize your own symptoms. It is much harder to transmit dormant virus, so the quicker you get treated, the less chance there is for you to pass the virus on to an unsuspecting partner.

Herpes

Herpes was *en vogue* in the late 1970s and early 1980s, achieving a certain cachet thanks to a flurry of media attention when rates of infection skyrocketed. Trendy magazines and news programs carried frequent stories while dating services sprang up to help infected individuals find each other. Although the media glare has definitely dimmed, infection rates have not. The Centers for Disease Control estimates that almost half a million new cases of genital herpes appear each year and that as many as 30 million Americans are infected. When all is said and done, one troubling fact remains: Once you have herpes, you have it for life.

For most of us, the word "herpes" conjures images of painful sores in sensitive spots, but herpes actually refers to a large group of viruses containing more than eighty subtypes. Most everyone has had a prior run-in with these common viruses—remember the chicken pox? You got that thanks to herpes zoster. A different type of herpes virus known as HHV-8 probably causes Kaposi's sarcoma in AIDS.

What we typically think of as a herpes infection is caused by two different types of the herpes simplex virus: herpes simplex type 1 (HSV-1) and herpes simplex type 2 (HSV-2). (Quite ingenious, isn't it?) It had been thought that HSV-1 caused infections above the belt line (most often on your mouth and lips) while HSV-2 caused them below the belt line. We now know this is not entirely the case; HSV-

2 can turn up in your mouth and, conversely, HSV-1 can infect your genitals.

The herpes simplex virus attacks only humans and is usually passed via direct sexual contact. Although doctors report sporadic transmission after close physical contact (particularly between patients and healthcare workers), unless you are a masseur, you can't get it from anything other than sex. The fact that herpes can infect your oral cavity is especially important if you enjoy fellatio. A condom would protect you, but most men don't use one unless ejaculation is planned. Just as you can catch herpes by sucking an infected penis—even if the herpes infection isn't currently active—the converse is also true: Your partner can spread the virus from his mouth to your penis.

Herpes passes to your anorectal region during rimming or unprotected rubbing of an infected partner's penis against your buttocks. Penetration is not necessary. Again, a condom would be protective, but most men use condoms only for penetration.

Once a herpes virus lands on your body, it invades the skin. You can't see the virus at this early stage, but you might notice symptoms that you associate with any viral illness, such as a low-grade fever, weakness, and an achy feeling. Within a week a burning sensation (occasionally quite painful) begins in the skin, followed, a day or two later, by a cluster of small, clear blisters. (See Figure 4.1.) Pain intensifies as blisters develop, and at this point you become highly contagious. You spread the virus not only to sexual partners but also to other parts of your own body (eyes, fingers, etc.). Do not touch your blisters, but if you do, wash your hands thoroughly with an antibacterial soap. As with chicken pox, blisters typically burst in three to five days, leaving shallow pink ulcers that crust over.

Once crusting is complete, healing without scarring occurs. The entire cycle usually lasts two weeks. Herpes then

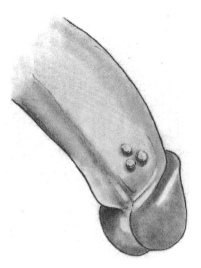

Figure 4.1: Herpes Blisters

enters a "latent phase" during which the virus goes into hiding. Although its exact location is unknown, doctors suspect the viruses hide in large sensory nerves around your sacrum. The virus remains dormant until something triggers it to reproduce and travel down the nerves to your anogenital region, where the cycle begins anew. Unfortunately, we do not know what triggers this change from latency to attack, and the length of time between outbreaks is completely unpredictable. Clearly, men with compromised immune systems (those with AIDS or on chemotherapy) are predisposed to recurrent attacks. Cancer or severe infections can precipitate an attack, as can local trauma to your anogenital region (especially sunburn, so keep those bathing suits on). Periods of intense emotional stress also have been associated with herpes outbreaks. Whatever the cause, most people experience another attack within a year after their initial infection. Expect four to five attacks in your first year, but some attacks can be so mild that you don't even know you're having one. Subsequent attacks are usually shorter, and healing occurs within one week. The good news is that over time, the frequency of outbreaks diminishes.

On the penis, herpes blisters occur anywhere, from the head and shaft to under your foreskin. (See Figure 4.1.) In your anal area, look for blisters on the surrounding skin or within the anus itself. If your anal canal or rectum is involved, symptoms typically include bleeding and intense pain during bowel movements. A bloody mucus discharge even without the passage of stool is common. The colon lining can become so inflamed that many times a herpes outbreak is misdiagnosed as colitis unless you are honest with your doctor and admit to having had anal sex.

It is often difficult for physicians to diagnose a herpes infection in your mouth, because blisters hide on the roof of your mouth or between your lips and gums. Symptoms are similar to what you would expect from any typical sore throat, with pain on swallowing, redness, and swollen lymph nodes (glands) in your neck. Because the blisters are tiny, your doctor can easily miss them. Unless you mention having had oral sex, most physicians won't even think of herpes and will dismiss you with instructions to take throat lozenges.

When herpes recurs in your mouth, it is usually at the edge of your lip and commonly is called a fever blister or cold sore. No matter how benign that name sounds, you still have a herpes infection that is highly contagious and easily passed to others.

To make the diagnosis of a herpes infection, doctors rely on a positive viral culture from your blister. Although this type of culture is done with a cotton swab, it differs markedly from typical bacterial cultures you may be used to. (Remember the strep test when your doctor rammed the long stick down your throat until you gagged?) A viral culture requires a different medium in which to grow, so if your doctor just performs a standard bacterial culture he or she will not find the herpes. The issue is further complicated by the fact that within two weeks your symptoms disappear on their own. This pattern is typical of any run-of-the-mill sore throat or nonspecific colitis, so the correct diagnosis is never made.

Why is it a problem if your herpes infection is missed, when it resolves on its own? First and foremost, failure to make the diagnosis allows you to unwittingly pass herpes on to other partners. Another advantage of making a timely diagnosis is that medications abort your attack.

In an untreated herpes outbreak, your immune system attacks the virus through a combination of antibodies and T-cells. Because your first episode sensitizes your immune system, subsequent attacks are shorter. Herpes antibodies can be detected in your blood and indicate that you've had a prior run-in with the virus. Patients with AIDS and low T-cell counts are prone to frequent and more severe recurrences.

Medications such as acyclovir (Zovirax) and its derivatives, valacyclovir (Valtrex) and famciclovir (Famvir), are available in tablet form by prescription. These drugs work to stop virus reproduction and typically shorten an attack. The standard dose of acyclovir for acute herpes outbreaks is either 200 milligrams (mg) five times a day or 400 mg three times a day for ten days. The latter dose is probably easier to manage and just as effective. Although valacyclovir is not approved by the Food and Drug Administration (FDA) for use in immunocompromised (AIDS) patients, most doctors find it effective. For first-time infections, the dose of valacyclovir is 1 gram twice a day for ten days, but with recurrent infections it decreases to 500 mg twice a day for five days. The recommended dose for famciclovir for acute attacks is 500 mg twice a day for seven days. Some physicians also recommend acyclovir cream in combination with pills, but many medical authorities feel that that provides little or no added benefit. These medications are relatively safe with few side effects and should be started at the first sign of an attack.

Men who have suffered through multiple prior herpes outbreaks generally can recognize their first symptoms (localized pain or burning in their anogenital region) and begin medication even before their blisters appear. Not only will this make their attack more tolerable by lessening pain and shortening its course, it also may decrease their chance of transmitting the virus to a partner.

People with HIV or severely compromised immune systems who suffer from repeated attacks may obtain relief by taking medications continuously. (See Chapter 5.) Called chronic suppression therapy, the standard dose of acyclovir is usually 800 mg daily but can be adjusted depending on immune status. The standard suppression dose of valacyclovir is 500 mg once a day; the dose for famciclovir is 125 mg twice a day. The extremely rare downside to chronic suppression is that herpes can become resistant to the common medications, and intravenous drugs will be required to fight outbreaks.

If you have herpes, it is best to inform all potential partners. Doctors used to think that you could transmit the virus only during outbreaks. Now we know transmission is possible, although less likely, even when you are symptom free. Clearly, abstinence at the first sign of a flare-up is key to preventing transmission and should continue until crusting is complete. If your anal canal is the only area infected, your penis is probably safe as long as your partner keeps his hands off your butt. Problems arise because many people are infected at multiple sites (penis, rectum, mouth, or in any combination).

No one wants to believe he has herpes, and I have had patients come into my office with painful sores attributed to everything from getting their penis caught in their zipper (wear underwear) to a partner's overzealous fellatio. When I tell patients they have herpes, most stare in disbelief, swearing that the penis they sucked or the ass they fucked was completely clean. That may be what they thought, but herpes blisters are hard to spot and easily hidden—especially in a partner's mouth and anus. Although the infection is usually painful and most people don't feel up to sex, attacks can be mild, and as blisters heal, pain abates but a partner can still infect you. Unfortunately, the herpes virus can be present without any symptoms, and your partner may not even know that he has it while he is passing the disease to you.

A common mistake men make (other than catching herpes in the first place) is assuming that a canker sore (aphthous ulcer) is herpes. Canker sores are usually solitary and covered with a white membrane; herpes blisters tend to be multiple and red once the blister pops. Canker sores affect different parts of your mouth with each outbreak and often are painless. A mild steroid cream applied directly to the ulcer speeds healing.

Molluscum Contagiosum

Molluscum contagiosum is not a shellfish but a sexually transmitted virus belonging to the pox family of viruses. Smallpox is also a member of this group, but thankfully, molluscum does not have the same grave prognosis. Molluscum contagiosum generally infects the skin, and in adults it is sexually transmitted through direct skin-to-skin contact. If your partner has the virus and you rub against an infected part of his body, chances are great that you'll catch it too. But as with herpes, transmission also has been reported after close nonsexual contact with an infected individual (massages, contact sports).

Approximately one to three months after exposure, molluscum causes a distinct pin-size pimple with a central depression (like a moon crater). (See Figure 4.2.) If left untreated, the sores gradually increase in size, sometimes reaching pea-size proportions. If you squeeze a sore, a cheesy white material oozes out. The lesions are often multiple and may not be clustered in one area. The most frequent sites of infection are the anogenital region with spread to your thighs and lower abdomen. It is also possible to spread the virus with your hands to more distant sites (arms, back, and face).

Molluscum typically produces few symptoms other than its characteristic skin lesions. If untreated, the virus runs its course within two to four months, but occasionally it per-

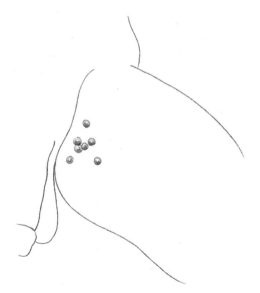

Figure 4.2: Molluscum Contagiosum

sists for years. If you think you have molluscum, see your physician, who can make the diagnosis with just a look. A biopsy is rarely necessary. Treatment will help you get rid of the unsightly skin ulcers faster and prevent spread to other parts of your body and to sexual partners.

Treatment for molluscum aims directly at the skin lesions. Oral and topical medications don't work, so the doctor must scrape, burn, or freeze the blisters away. (Don't worry, it doesn't hurt.) If treatment becomes painful, a bit of local anesthesia is more than adequate. Catching molluscum early is key (especially for men with HIV) before the virus multiplies and soon you have sores everywhere. In men with AIDS, neglected molluscum can become impossible to cure.

Skin lesions also can become secondarily infected with bacteria (usually staphylococcus), and then antibiotics are necessary. Bacterial infection also increases the likelihood of scarring. It is crucial that you be checked periodically for two to three months after treatment. Doctors can treat only visible skin blisters, leaving behind virus at other sites that has not grown into the characteristic lesions. Repeat checkups rid you of these viruses as soon as lesions appear and reduce your risk of another major infection.

Although molluscum has not been shown to enter a dormant state like herpes, recurrences are seen. We don't know whether recurrence represents a new infection or reactivation of molluscum from within the cell.

Condyloma Acuminatum

My patient narrowed his eyes in anger. I had just told him he had anal warts. "So Billy's cheating on me," he said.

I took a deep breath. "No, it doesn't mean that at all."

"Well, I know I'm not cheating on him, so who else is there?"

"No one," I said. "These warts are caused by viruses. Billy

72

could have carried it for years—from long before the two of you got together.''

"Even without his having anything on his penis?" I nodded, and his face brightened for a moment. "Are you just saying that so I don't kill him when I get home?''

Condyloma acuminatum (also called venereal warts or genital warts) are caused by the human papillomavirus (HPV). As the name "venereal" implies, the virus spreads from partner to partner during sex. The Centers for Disease Control estimates that close to 1 million new HPV infections occur each year, with more than 24 million Americans already infected. Gay men with healthy sex lives are finding it increasingly difficult to avoid condyloma. It is estimated that more than half of all HIV-negative men who have sex with men carry the virus, and the number increases to almost 100 percent for HIV-positive men. Unfortunately, you can carry HPV and infect sex partners without knowing you have it. We don't know why at times the virus grows into a wart and other times it does not.

As with other viral STDs we have discussed, transmission between partners can occur without penetration or ejaculation. Your partner's unprotected penis rubbing between your buttocks during seemingly innocuous foreplay is more than enough. Even if he wears a condom, the base of his shaft, scrotum, and pubic region are not covered (unless he's inside a plastic bag), and these are frequent sites for warts that rub against you during sex. Read on, it gets worse. The type of HPV responsible for venereal warts does not grow on hands, but a hand can carry the virus between sex partners or to another location on your own body. Dildos and other toys can also transmit virus between partners.

I have had patients swear that they have never allowed anyone close to their anus and yet they still got anal condyloma. (Are they lying?) HPV does not always grow into warts, especially on a penis. You touch his penis during sex and transport the virus to your anus the next time you wipe. (So always wash your hands.)

There are close to one hundred different numbered types of HPV, and although many cause genital warts, others cause different conditions, from hand and plantar warts, to laryngeal cancer. Some types of HPV (type 16 and 18) are associated with anogenital cancers (cervical in women and anal in men).

Most patients I see are afraid to admit they have condyloma because it makes them feel dirty and cheap. Instead, they come to my office complaining of hemorrhoids and are shocked when I tell them they have venereal warts. I must say right now that you are not cheap, and you are not dirty. (Or maybe I just don't you well enough.) The human papillomavirus is everywhere, and it may be next to impossible for an unattached gay man to have an active, *healthy* sex life and keep from getting condyloma. It is far easier to transmit HPV than HIV during sex.

So many common misconceptions surround condyloma that I must dispel them before going on.

❖ The type of human papillomavirus that causes condyloma is not the same type that causes hand warts. It is possible to spread condyloma to other warm, moist parts of your body (under your breasts, armpits, mouth), but it is extremely rare to find them on your fingers. You did not get venereal warts because some guy you were with had garden-variety hand warts.

❖ Although there have been isolated reports, you did not catch warts from a toilet seat or sauna. (Unless, of course, you did more in there than soak up the steam.)

❖ Straight men get anal warts too. I once had the father of an obviously closeted gay teen storm into my office demanding to know how his "all-American" son got "those things." Clearly the father was afraid the warts meant his son was gay, and his son was positively apoplectic over the idea that his father would learn the truth. Well, I'm a surgeon, not a shrink, so I explained to the father that just because his son had warts did not mean he was gay. Straight men are into butt play (the father nodded knowingly), and fingers can transmit the virus during hetero sex. Men can also self-infect themselves from penis to anus. Both father and son left smiling, but, as always, I caution you to be honest with your doctor and admit to anal sex so he or she can evaluate you properly.

◈ The wart is not the actual virus. It is your skin's reaction to the virus within it.

Typically, Condyloma acuminatum appears on your anogenital region, including your penis, anus, scrotum, pubic region, inner thighs, buttocks, and anal canal. The time between the virus landing on your body and the appearance of your wart is very variable, lasting anywhere from six weeks to eight months and occasionally as long as years. Most doctors believe the average incubation period is about three months, but keep in mind that the virus doesn't always grow into a wart. This becomes a major issue for gay men in monogamous relationships when partners automatically assume that the presence of warts on one means cheating. Well, don't assume anything. Just because warts turned up now doesn't mean that you just caught the virus. It could have been hanging out on your body for years, put there by one of your *previous* boyfriends. Even after warts have been completely destroyed, the virus may remain dormant in your cells. Some doctors believe you never get rid of HPV, and any recurrence represents a reactivation of virus you already had, not a new infection. And before you accuse your partner of cheating, look in the mirror. You could have brought the virus to him! Just because a wart didn't grow on you doesn't mean you're free of HPV.

Unlike the uniform appearance of molluscum, condyloma can all look very different. They vary from a whitish color to a shade lighter (hypopigmented) or darker (hyperpigmented) than your normal skin. (See Figure 4.3.) Most are raised and resemble tiny bunches of cauliflower, while others appear more like dark skin blemishes. If you find one wart, you can bet you have others in various stages of development. I have seen warts neglected for so long that they cover the man's entire buttocks. At this stage they usually have a foul order and ooze a purulent (infected) fluid. I am always stunned when I ask a patient why he didn't come in sooner and he answers, "But I just noticed this."

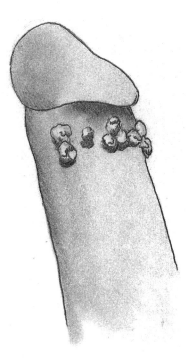

Figure 4.3: Condyloma Acuminatum

Although warts often cause itching, the most common first symptom is the wart itself. It gradually increases in size and others appear. If you have anal warts, rectal bleeding and pain after bowel movements and anal sex are other common complaints. Occasionally an anal wart creates a painful fissure that fails to heal without surgery. Warts on your penis probably won't cause any symptoms at all. Although unsightly if they grow large, they aren't painful and rarely bleed. Penile warts can spread down your urethra (the tube that carries urine through your penis) and cause bleeding or burning with urination.

So you think you've got them; now what do you do? See your physician immediately. A diagnosis often can be made visually, and biopsy is seldom necessary. Don't be startled if your doctor wraps a gauze soaked in vinegar around your penis or places it against your anus. Vinegar (acetic acid) turns warts white and helps your physician identify them. Which brings me to another important point: All bumps on your penis or anus are not warts. Hair follicles are often raised. If you suspect a wart and routinely shave your genitals, stop, because shaving inflames hair follicles and makes the diagnosis more difficult. Skin tags are also commonly found in this area but bear no relation to warts. They do not need to be removed unless you find them unsightly. So relax and let your doctor put on the acetic acid. It won't hurt, the acid is very dilute.

If you have warts around your anus, be sure your physician inserts a small lighted scope (anoscope) into your anus and looks on the inside as well. Don't be frightened, the scope is less than six inches long and not very thick. Discomfort is minimal and the exam takes less than a minute. If your doctor says it isn't necessary or can't perform this simple test (many dermatologists and internists don't have the capability in their offices), find one who will. What is visible on the outside of your anus is usually just the tip of the iceberg; you probably have many more warts on the inside. If your doctor only treats your external warts, they will continue to recur. Each time you move your bowels you push human papillomavirus out with your feces and reinfect your skin.

I have had patients refuse anoscopy saying "You don't have to look inside because nothing has ever gone up there." Wrong! Each time you wipe after a bowel movement, fingers and toilet paper gently probe your opening, and virus can easily be pushed inside. Other patients argue that they couldn't possibly have warts because they've checked their partners thoroughly. Unfortunately, just because you don't see a wart doesn't mean he isn't carrying the virus. Warts are five to ten times more common in the anal canals of gay men than on their penises. No one knows what stimulates a virus to blossom into a wart, but we do know that it grows better in the moist anal area than on a penis. Consequently, virus from your partner's penis where a wart *doesn't* grow gets transmitted to your anal area where it does grow.

So you have warts; now what do you do? Have them removed. If you don't, they will continue to grow, spread to others, and possibly change to cancers. *Do not treat warts yourself with over-the-counter preparations meant for hands!* In case you haven't noticed, your penis is not your finger. Venereal warts are more numerous than typical hand warts—especially in your anus—and you cannot do a thorough job. Putting caustic lotions meant for hands into your anus can be very dangerous.

I know you want to tell me that you've heard of cases of warts disappearing on their own. That's true; there are *isolated* reports in the medical literature of spontaneous regression of condyloma, but the incidence is rare. All I can say is: "Don't count on it. See your doctor."

Treatments available for condyloma through your doctor

are numerous and varied. Which one is best? The only way to answer this frequently asked question is to repeat what a physician friend of mine always says: "If one treatment was unequivocally better than the others there wouldn't be so many alternatives available." When a report in the medical literature proclaims one treatment as best, it isn't long before another contradicts those same results. The following are the most common procedures and medications available through your physician. Familiarize yourself with them so you can discuss the pros and cons of each before settling on a course of action.

TOPICAL AGENTS Topical medications have long been the mainstay of condyloma therapy. In essence, a caustic cream or liquid applied directly to a wart erodes it layer by layer. Podocon-25 (podophyllin), manufactured from a plant resin, is the most common medication in this class and was first used to treat condyloma in the 1940s. Your doctor dabs it on your warts, and you wash it off twelve hours later. Podophyllin will burn surrounding skin unless applied carefully and requires reapplication every one to two weeks until the wart completely disappears. Scarring rarely occurs.

Trichloroacetic acid is another common topical agent many doctors use. Like podophyllin, it's applied weekly until your wart disappears but has the added advantage of not needing to be washed off. Both agents irritate normal skin if not used carefully. A slight burning sensation after application is common but quickly passes. While small warts may go away with just one treatment, larger warts can require repeated applications over weeks or even months.

Podofilox (Condylox) is available by prescription and, unlike the other two medications, it is designed for home use. Apply it to external warts only, twice daily for three days, followed by a four-day rest. Repeat the cycle each week until your warts disappear, but be sure your doctor monitors your progress.

Topical medications are best used on penile warts, which are usually isolated and easily identified. Recurrence is rare when treatment continues until the wart completely disappears. If penile warts keep coming back after *complete* resolution, see a urologist. You may have warts inside your urethra that keep seeding the outside skin.

Although some physicians recommend caustic topical agents for perianal warts, I usually advise against it. Perianal warts in gay men, as mentioned earlier, are usually just the tip of the iceberg; the most advanced lesions are inside the anal canal. Although these medications can cure warts outside your anus, don't expect the cure to last. Untreated warts inside your anal canal will continually reinfect your perianal skin. Some doctors think that just swabbing your anal canal blindly with a topical agent is enough to destroy internal condyloma. No such luck. Your rectal lining is folded like a pie crust, so each fold must be spread open to expose hidden warts. Random application inside your anus and rectum misses some warts while burning completely normal areas. Topical agents applied within your anus and rectum also can cause severe pain and a bloody rectal discharge.

What do you do if after a thorough internal examination your doctor is positive all your warts are on the outside? Try topical agents, but watch closely to be sure your warts don't come back.

IMMUNOTHERAPY This class of medications stimulates your body's own defenses to destroy your warts. Immunotherapy is relatively new and carried out under your doctor's supervision. Interferon is a chemical manufactured by human white blood cells that helps fight various infections. Your doctor injects genetically engineered interferon directly into a wart. Interferon has many side effects (including high fevers, shaking chills, "flulike" symptoms) that limit its use to only five warts at a time. Most physicians use interferon only in men who have failed less toxic treatments (podophyllin, surgery, etc.). The doctor injects the medication twice weekly into the base of the wart until it disappears, or for a maximum of eight weeks. Because there are so many other less toxic treatments available, interferon should be viewed as a last resort.

Imiquimod (Aldara Cream 5%) is a physician-prescribed topical immunotherapy medication you can use in the privacy of your home. Although we don't know exactly how imiquimod destroys warts, it seems to stimulate people's own natural immunity. It works better in women than men, but in men it destroys penile warts faster than it works for perianal disease. Men with AIDS and low T-cell counts (less than 150) should not use the medication. Apply imiquimod to external warts only (don't push it up into your anus) at bedtime three times a week and wash it off in the morning. Skin reddening and irritation are common side effects that clear up if you skip an extra day between treatments. Your warts should disappear within four months; lengthier therapy is not recommended.

SURGERY Numerous surgical procedures to destroy venereal warts have evolved over the years, encompassing everything from the cold steel of scalpels to the high tech of lasers. Surgeons can cut out warts or use extreme temperatures to rapidly freeze or burn them away; most often they use a combination of techniques. Surgery works best for patients who have failed other treatments, have large bulky warts that would take too long to dissolve with topical agents, or have warts within their hard-to-treat anal canal. Although more painful than other treatments, surgery has its advantages: All the warts are destroyed in a single sitting

81

(or lying, as the case may be) and a piece is sent for biopsy to check for cancer.

Some of the following treatments may not sound like surgery, but they all require some form of anesthesia. If your warts are small and isolated, local anesthesia may be enough, but if extensive or inside your anorectal canal, more complete relaxation is needed. Some doctors can remove even the most extensive anal warts safely in their offices, but most often you'll need a trip to an operating room at a hospital or ambulatory surgery center. (An overnight stay is rarely required.)

Surgeons use scalpels and scissors to cut out warts and send them to a pathologist, who checks for cancer. After removing some warts for biopsy, most surgeons then switch to destroying the bulk of the warts with high heat from electric current (cautery) or freezing them away with liquid nitrogen. Extreme temperatures have the advantage of killing warts with very little bleeding, but to prevent recurrence, the entire wart must be destroyed.

Some surgeons also use lasers to eradicate warts. The frequently used carbon dioxide laser beam hits a wart with energy from its invisible light and instantly heats it to the boiling point. The wart goes up in a cloud of smoke with very little injury to surrounding healthy tissue. Physicians who advocate this technique of laser vaporization report faster healing with a lower incidence of wart recurrence over other standard surgical methods.

No matter what treatment method your doctor employs, be sure he or she uses acetic acid to bring out the tiniest warts that might otherwise be missed. A missed wart guarantees you'll be back for more treatment, and neither you nor your doctor wants that. If you have external anal warts, your surgeon must carefully dilate your sphincter to check inside for hidden warts.

Whether your warts are burned, frozen, or cut away,

don't be surprised when your surgeon doesn't sew up the hole left behind. To prevent infection, the skin is left open so healing occurs from the inside out. While tiny warts heal quickly, large open areas from bulky warts often take weeks to fill in. Taking frequent baths to keep your wounds clean prevents infection and speeds healing.

Unfortunately, most gay men know someone who has been surgically treated for anal warts—someone who all too willingly recounts the horrors of his postoperative period. Sadly, these men are not exaggerating when they describe hours soaking in the tub (sitz bath) moaning with pain. Gay men often put off treatment until they are walking around with an asshole that looks like it's been hung with Christmas tree ornaments. They have so many warts that any surgical procedure becomes extensive. And afterward, their open wounds discharge a bloody fluid that stains their underwear.

If you need surgery, be sure your physician gives you adequate pain medication. (A narcotic is often required.) While you won't be pain free (for that you'd have to be in a coma), you should be fairly comfortable. In short, expect a week of hell. The only way to avoid it is to see your doctor at the first sign of condyloma. The quicker you're treated, the less chance there is for spread.

Some surgeons advise a series of surgeries for advanced cases, removing a little each time. I am opposed to this practice, because mini-treatments are no less painful and the process is spread out over many weeks. Also, while one area is treated, it can become reinfected from another. Bite the bullet, bend over, and get it done all at once.

Wart recurrence is a major problem, no matter what the treatment. Even after radical surgery aimed at total elimination of anorectal condyloma, expect a recurrence rate of up to 50 percent, with 20 to 30 percent being average. Fortunately, subsequent treatments don't have to be as bad as your first. Most recurrences, if caught early, are handled with a simple "touch-up" in the doctor's office with topical agents. Don't keep putting it off until your warts have multiplied and you're right back where you started.

Patients with HIV are more prone to extensive warts that recur more often. Unfortunately, HIV treatment alone will not make warts disappear. If you have HIV and suspect venereal warts (most patients with HIV also harbor the human papillomavirus), seek treatment immediately. This is not something that will go away, and, in all likelihood, it will get worse very quickly. And don't assume that just because you see doctors for HIV, they also check you for warts (or any other STD) regularly. If you feel something, tell your doctor about it and be sure it's looked at.

ANAL CANCER It may seem absurd to include anal cancer under the global heading of STDs, but more and more scientific data support just this conclusion. Anal cancer is neither the typical colon cancer nor the Kaposi's sarcoma common in AIDS. Anal cancer is a squamous cell tumor that closely resembles cervical cancer in women. Squamous cells, as you may recall from Chapter 2, line your anus and are similar to skin cells found elsewhere on your body. Your anal lining ends with a series of glands at the dentate line. (See Figure 2.1.) These glands are analogous to those found in a woman's cervix, and doctors have long known that cervical cancer is directly related to infection with certain types of human papillomavirus. The many varieties of HPV are numbered; types 16 and 18 predispose you to cancer, whereas types 6 and 11 cause warts. The same virus can infect a woman's cervix and your anus. Unfortunately, most HPV infections contain multiple types, so you end up with warts as well as dangerous areas progressing toward cancer.

Before the HIV epidemic, the incidence of anal cancer

in gay men who had anoreceptive intercourse was equal to the rates of cervical cancer in women before the advent of Pap smears. In the AIDS era we have seen a dramatic increase in anal cancer in men who have sex with men. It is now the fourth most common malignancy associated with HIV. Frightening? You bet, but it doesn't have to be.

From the comprehensive study of cervical cancer, doctors know that squamous cell cancer progresses through various stages whereby normal cells infected with HPV gradually change into cancerous cells. The various stages in this transformation can be seen with a microscope. For years women have routinely gone for a Pap smear, in which a swab is used to pick up samples of their cervical cells for microscopic examination. Mildly abnormal cells are called low grade dysplasia; severely abnormal cells (potentially malignant) are high grade dysplasia.

In order to obtain a sample of your anal cells for cytologic examination (a Pap smear), the doctor passes a Dacron swab into your anus. Abnormal cells stick to the swab, and the doctor can transfer them to a microscope slide. Although lubricant cannot be used because it distorts cells, the Dacron swab is small and causes minimal discomfort. Unfortunately, a Pap smear is still not a routine part of most medical evaluations. If your doctor doesn't do one, ask for it.

Low grade dysplasia carries little risk of underlying malignancy, but high grade dysplasia is a more serious threat. Although the study of anal dysplasia is just beginning, given the cervical cancer model, many doctors believe that high grade dysplasia has a significant risk of progressing to an invasive cancer. Men with HIV have a higher risk for developing high grade dysplasia that progresses to invasive cancer than do those who are HIV negative.

HIV-negative men who have anoreceptive intercourse should obtain a Pap smear once a year, and HIV-positive men should have it twice a year. If normal cells are found, nothing further needs to be done. Low grade dysplasia might mean underlying condyloma or cells in the early stages of transformation to cancer. Low grade dysplasia doesn't always progress to high grade, and the cells can return to normal. Obviously a Pap smear with low grade changes needs to be followed with repeat examinations at six- to twelve-month intervals.

When women have abnormal Pap smears, their gynecologist does a colposcopy and checks the cervix with a microscope. Under magnification, abnormal areas of dysplasia look different from normal counterparts. The gynecologist can then sample these areas for cancer. Surgeons are just beginning to apply colposcopy to men with dysplasia.

If your doctor tells you that you have high grade dysplasia, don't automatically assume that you have a deadly cancer. For cancer to be lethal, its cells must be more than malignant, they must also have the ability to spread. This ability to spread is the last step in evolution for any cancer and cannot be determined through a Pap smear. You need to have a biopsy where a tiny piece of anal lining is snipped out (it doesn't hurt) and sent to the lab to be studied. The pathologist looks at an entire cluster of cells and determines if there is any sign of invasion (the ability to spread). If there is, then you have a true cancer, and chemotherapy and radiation may be required. When only dysplasia is present without any sign of invasion, simple excision of all abnormal tissue is treatment enough. Your doctor needs to use a microscope to magnify your anal glands to find these tiny areas that typically don't look like warts. If your surgeon just treats your warts, dangerous areas of dysplasia may be left behind.

Hepatitis

Hepatitis is a viral infection of the liver caused by several different types of viruses. The most common are hepatitis

A, B, and C. Although hepatitis D, E, and G also have been identified, they are rare. I include hepatitis as an STD because, for many men who have sex with men, the virus passes between partners during sex. The word "hepatitis" fills most of us with dread, but often the virus, no matter what type, causes an asymptomatic infection (you don't know you have it) that goes away on its own. The only indication that you ever had the disease comes when your doctor tells you blood tests showed you're immune to future infections.

Hepatitis can, on rare occasions, take a much more dangerous course and, instead of a mild infection, progress to liver failure and death. Other times the infection improves but never quite goes away (chronic hepatitis), and the virus slowly, over many years, destroys your liver. Fortunately, liver failure occurs in less than 1 percent of infections, but chronic hepatitis can be much more common and depends on the type of infecting virus. Chronic hepatitis may eventually lead to cirrhosis or liver cancer.

When first infected with hepatitis, you feel fine—but the virus continues to multiply, destroying more and more liver cells. Your urine darkens to tea color and the whites of your eyes turn yellow as jaundice begins. Profound weakness and fatigue set in, along with loss of appetite, nausea, and vomiting. Many men feel like they can't even get out of bed. Smokers complain that cigarettes have lost their taste—a strong indication that they may have hepatitis. Doctors diagnose hepatitis through blood tests, which identify either the virus or the antibodies made to fight the infection.

HEPATITIS A Hepatitis A is often called infectious hepatitis, but this is really a misnomer because all forms of hepatitis are infectious. Hepatitis A is frequently passed via a fecal-oral route. Sound disgusting? A common way for many diseases to spread, fecal-oral contamination does not imply that you've eaten an infected person's shit (although always beware of rimming!). People can transmit the virus from their stool to your mouth when they don't wash their hands before preparing food. (Now you know why your mother always told you to wash!) Clams and other shellfish also can ingest hepatitis virus in contaminated water and pass it when you enjoy those raw bar delicacies.

Although you certainly feel sick, hepatitis A is rarely fatal and does not progress to a chronic condition. You become infectious at the end of an incubation period (approximately two to six weeks)—even before you know you're sick. During this dangerous time you can unwittingly pass the virus to other people, even through kissing. You remain infectious until your antibody levels rise high enough to contain and then kill the virus. In most cases the disease runs its course within six to eight weeks and your liver recovers completely.

To prevent infecting household members, separate your dishes from theirs, washing everything thoroughly. Hand washing after a bowel movement is, of course, crucial, but self-isolation is not. If you lock yourself away, you'll only feel more depressed, and this will worsen your condition. You need someone around to cheer you up, push you to eat when food has no taste, and dispense that all-important bit of TLC. Stories detail ridiculous extremes people go to trying to protect themselves from hepatitis: One man drained his pool because a friend recovering from hepatitis went for an uninvited swim, and another threw out every dish his lover touched before they switched to paper.

HEPATITIS B AND C Before HIV, hepatitis B was probably the most dangerous viral infection gay men faced. Hepatitis C is a relatively newly identified virus and most often causes post-transfusion hepatitis. Although two different viruses, many of their characteristics are similar. Both are passed between partners in semen, blood, and other bodily fluids and both have significant risk for becoming chronic. Unlike hepatitis A, hepatitis B and C can, in less than 1 percent of cases, progress to liver failure and death. The incubation period between infection and the appearance of symptoms ranges from two weeks to six months, and like hepatitis A, most men are infectious before they realize they have the disease.

For men with HIV, hepatitis B and C can be lethal. They are more likely to enter a state of chronic infection with progressive liver destruction. Hepatitis B becomes chronic in less than 2 percent of men with normal immune systems, but if HIV is present, 90 percent of infections become chronic. Hepatitis C is far more dangerous and becomes chronic in 90 percent of men with *normal* immune systems, and 20 percent eventually develop cirrhosis.

Isolation is not required to prevent transmission of hepatitis B or C, but safe-sex practices are a must. Many physicians advise abstinence until your hepatitis resolves.

HEPATITIS TREATMENTS No specific drugs treat acute hepatitis. See your doctor regularly so that your liver function and nutritional status can be monitored. If nausea is a problem, try eating bigger meals in the morning, since nausea tends to worsen throughout the day. In severe cases, doctors prescribe medications to stop your vomiting. Intravenous fluids might be necessary. Rest is crucial. Occasionally hospitalization is required for closer monitoring and nutritional support. Stay away from steroids, which are of no benefit and may even be harmful.

Avoid drugs and alcohol, which further tax your liver, until you're *fully* recovered. This may seem intuitive, but I have seen men who notice their eyes are no longer yellow and assume they're cured. They've been out of circulation for too long and venture outside for a bit of fresh air—only to end up in a bar toasting their recovery. The next morning their eyes are yellow again! Not a good thing.

If hepatitis virus persists in your blood for more than six months, you probably have a chronic infection. Most doctors will advise a liver biopsy followed by a course of interferon injections. Although the side effects can be severe, interferon provides the best chance of eliminating or alleviating the chronic infection. In HIV-negative men, interferon is more successful in treating hepatitis B than C. Never embark on interferon therapy without a thorough understanding of its many risks and benefits.

IMMUNIZATION Like many other viral illnesses, immunization against some forms of hepatitis is now available. Immunization falls into two categories: that which prevents infection immediately after exposure and that which delivers long-lasting protection. Immune globulin contains antibodies against either hepatitis A or B (so be sure you get the right one); getting the injection immediately after exposure to an infected person will usually prevent you from contracting the disease. One patient I had refused immunization, saying, "I'll take my chances because I don't want to get AIDS from the shot." This is an old queens' tale, because immune globulin poses no risk of AIDS transmission.

Immunization providing lasting immunity to either hepatitis A or B is also available, and again it is type specific. For hepatitis A, a single injection provides immunity to most men with minor side effects (a sore arm). A booster shot administered six to twelve months after the primary inoculation heightens your immunity.

Hepatitis B vaccine is genetically engineered so your risk of developing acute hepatitis from it is zero. Low-grade fever and a sore arm are the most frequent complaints. You'll need three vaccinations spread over six months.

90

Over 95 percent of people who receive all three shots become immune, and a booster is recommended at one year. If you are exposed to hepatitis B and have not had a prior immunization, you should receive both immune globulin and vaccine.

Men who have sex with men should receive prophylactic immunization against both hepatitis A and B—unless a prior infection already has left them immune. Unfortunately, there is no vaccine available against hepatitis C.

Summary

HIV is not the only viral sexually transmitted disease. Most are far more prevalent *and* far more contagious than HIV. Safe sex may not protect you from them, and they may not be curable.

- Be honest with your doctor.
- Once you are infected, the virus may be in your body for life.
- Seek treatment at the first sign of an outbreak.
- If you have one STD, chances are you have another.
- Just because you see your doctor for HIV doesn't mean that you've been checked for other STDs.
- Do not treat venereal warts yourself with over-the-counter medications.
- Get a Pap smear.
- Get vaccinated against hepatitis.

CHAPTER 5

HIV—

STILL DEADLY AFTER

ALL THESE YEARS

A *young man, still in his twenties, sits before me. We're separated by my desk, but he seems miles away. He shifts in his chair, and his smile droops at the corners. I've been taking care of him for close to a decade. I thumb through his records—eight tests and all negative. I can't stall any longer, so I take a deep breath and shatter his world.*

"This time your test was positive." There, I've said it.

His smile stays frozen, and only his watery eyes tell me he's heard. I point to the box of tissues, but he shakes his head.

"I've kind of been expecting it," he says finally. "I mean, it was just a matter of time."

He's so wrong.

In 1981 growing numbers of gay men arrived at emergency rooms in New York and California with *Pneumocystis carinii* pneumonia (PCP), a disease doctors rarely saw. Whether called gay-related immune deficiency (GRID) or by any of the other early names attached to it, AIDS had arrived. Although it wasn't until 1983 that the human immunodeficiency virus (HIV) was finally identified, scientific evidence points to its presence in this country as early as 1978.

In 1985 the Food and Drug Administration licensed the first test to detect HIV, but it wasn't until 1987 that zidovudine (AZT, or Retrovir) became the first drug approved specifically for AIDS treatment. Until then available medications treated only the infections and cancers that HIV allowed to proliferate. So many milestones in a disease not even identified twenty years ago, but for most it has seemed like a lifetime.

The World Health Organization (WHO) estimates that, worldwide, over 30 million people had HIV at the end of 1997 and, if trends continue, by the new millennium, 60 to 70 million adults will carry HIV, with 90 percent of them living in Third World countries. Already in some African countries 25 percent of adults carry the virus. To date, more than 60 percent of those with HIV have died. In the United States, over 600,000 cases of AIDS have been reported to the Centers for Disease Control, and more than 50 percent of these infections occurred in men who have had sex with men. This number, however, is falling while rates for heterosexual transmission are rising. The Centers for Disease Control estimates that more than 40,000 to 80,000 new HIV infections occur in the United States each year. Most recent data give New York City the dubious distinction of having the most cases of AIDS, with Los Angeles coming in second. Even with all we have learned over the years about safe-sex practices and the advent of new drugs, HIV is still prevalent and deadly.

This chapter is an overview of HIV, its treatment and prospects for the future. It is not a substitute for a conversation with your doctor. Although the information presented is current, HIV treatment changes almost daily. What you read today may not hold true several months from now. Because of the rapid advances in the field, I urge you to be tested regularly—especially if your sexual practices place you at risk—and see a physician the moment you test positive. HIV is not something that will go away if you ignore it.

The key to living a long and healthy life depends as much on your efforts as on medications. Find a doctor whose practice is largely devoted to HIV, because treatment is complicated and should not be left to someone who sees only a few cases each year. Those of us who treat AIDS still see patients ravaged by disease begging for help. They come to us as a last hope, after years of being treated by some doctor watching viral loads rise and T-cells fall while telling them there is no real treatment for this virus. While there is no specific medical specialty in AIDS treatment, most physicians working in the field are internal medicine specialists with a special interest in the disease. (See Chapter 12.)

When I tell most patients they have HIV, their eyes close as they recall "that time" they messed up. Most want to talk about it, as if admission lessens their guilt. They speak in half-thoughts of memories suddenly too painful to bear. This young man was no different. He bit his lower lip and shook his head while I waited for him to speak. "He'd only rub it on the outside. He promised . . . but then it was on the inside—it felt too good. I tried to say something, but his kisses swallowed my words."

"You were too afraid he'd leave," I said.

His eyes widened as if he suddenly understood. "He promised he wouldn't come."

The guy lied.

Every HIV-positive man has an excuse why he let down his guard. After years of preaching the importance of safe sex, gay men still contract the virus. Perhaps it was the Ecstacy or alcohol that made you drop your guard. Or maybe you're just sick of those condoms. Many men allow unprotected sex because they're too afraid they'll lose the hottest guy they've ever had if they ask him to put on a condom. I am always angered when someone tells me that safe sex is such a "bother" and doesn't really matter—now that the protease inhibitors practically cure the disease. Sadly, this is not the case.

The Virus

There are two types of human immunodeficiency viruses: HIV-1 and HIV-2. HIV-1 causes most of the cases of AIDS in the United States, with only isolated HIV-2 infections reported. The virus is a retrovirus and contains RNA instead of DNA as its genetic code. For infection to occur, the virus must get into your bloodstream and bind to a protein receptor on your lymphocyte. (It's like a little landing pad.) But it cannot infect just any lymphocyte. HIV specifically targets CD4+ lymphocytes, which are a type of T-cell. Once firmly attached to the T-cell, the virus injects its RNA into the cell. In humans, our genetic building block is DNA, not RNA. An enzyme called reverse transcriptase converts HIV RNA into DNA. This newly formed virus DNA passes into your cell's nucleus and links up with your own DNA. Then viral DNA commandeers its host's reproductive machinery, issuing a command to manufacture more copies of virus DNA. At this point your CD4+ lymphocyte has been converted into an HIV factory. Besides manufacturing viral DNA that gets changed back into RNA, your lymphocyte also builds protein coats to cover the HIV RNA. After each new virus is fully assembled, it leaves the CD4+ cell to infect other T-cells.

Sound complicated? For sure, but it is also a highly efficient process producing an estimated 10 billion copies of HIV each day. Medications combat HIV by blocking any number of these steps in reproduction. Most HIV does not circulate in your bloodstream; instead it remains hidden in T-lymphocytes and lymph nodes.

Your immune system fights back by manufacturing antibodies that attack the HIV, but they can't wipe out the infection. Most HIV tests measure these antibodies. A positive test indicates infection. In three weeks to six months antibodies appear and virus levels in your blood fall. The disease then enters its clinically "latent" phase when most men feel fine, but their CD4+ lymphocytes are gradually being destroyed. After approximately ten years without treatment, CD4+ counts fall below 200. With increasing suppression of your immune system, HIV proliferates and your viral load (a measure of virus particles in your bloodstream) rises. It is at this point that AIDS develops.

HIV is not that easy to catch. The virus spreads through blood or bodily fluids (semen and possibly saliva). Gay men are infected most often through unprotected anal sex (ejaculation is not required) or intravenous drug use with shared needles. You may be thinking that you've never shot drugs, but how about steroids? Ever share a needle for that? The virus doesn't care if it gets into your body on a coke, heroin, or steroid ride.

Although some researchers report isolated cases of HIV transmission through oral sex, the risk is far lower. (See Chapter 9.) Open cuts on fingers or in your mouth or anus make infection more likely. Concomitant STDs, including herpes and gonorrhea, also make it easier for you to catch HIV, probably by creating small sores through which the virus gains access to your bloodstream. The opposite is also true. If your HIV-positive partner has another STD he becomes more infective, probably because his viral load rises with infection and increased penile inflammation allows even more virus into his semen. A multitude of other factors, including your health and your partner's viral load, also influences your chances of being infected. Although I have seen statistics estimating that the average person needs twenty unprotected sexual encounters to contract HIV, I wouldn't bet on it. Having unprotected sex with the idea that you probably won't catch HIV even if your partner has it is like Russian roulette—you never know which shot has the bullet.

Although much has been made about the risk of transmission between an HIV-positive physician and his or her patient, to date there is only one suspected case in the United States of HIV passing from a doctor to a patient: the Florida dentist who transmitted HIV to his female patient. The risk of infection for healthcare workers stuck with a needle from an HIV-positive patient is far less than 1 percent. Blood transfusion is another area where risk has dropped significantly with the advent of routine donor screening.

HIV Testing

The ELISA (enzyme-linked immunosorbent assay) test checks for viral antibodies in blood and is the mainstay of HIV testing. Although very accurate, there are occasional false positive results among patients with chronic diseases, such as hepatitis and collagen vascular diseases (lupus). For this reason, every test is repeated on the same sample of blood with the more specific Western blot test. If this is also positive, you have HIV.

Confirmation of HIV antibodies by a second test before telling patients they have HIV had been the standard in this country to protect those few individuals who have a positive ELISA but negative Western blot test. These patients do not have HIV but could be told they do after just one test. In medicine, we routinely use phrases like "It looks like it's cancer" or "You probably have an infection" for many other illnesses before definite confirmation; not with HIV—until now.

In March 1998 the Centers for Disease Control reversed its previous long-standing policy of recommending two test confirmations of HIV before patients were told. Now the Centers for Disease Control advocates an HIV test called the Murex rapid test, which provides results in as little as ten minutes. This test also checks for HIV antibodies. Positive results should be confirmed by Western blot, which usually takes an extra day. Patients who test positive by rapid test are told that they are "probably" HIV positive but that another confirmatory test is needed. The Centers for Disease Control reversed its policy because nearly 700,000 people take the HIV ELISA blood test each year but never return for their results. It is hoped that patients will wait while rapid tests are performed. Rapid tests also save patients from up to a week of needless anxiety while they wait for results by standard methods. On the downside, some doctors do not agree with the Centers for Disease Control and worry that the rapid test is less accurate than the ELISA.

If a needle stick scares you, an OraSure test checks a sample of your oral secretions (not saliva) for HIV antibodies. The test is as accurate as blood tests, and results are available in anywhere from three to seven days. The downside is that most facilities do not have the capability to perform the OraSure.

No matter which test you choose, be sure to ask when you will have results. They should take no more than two to three days. Don't submit to testing by anyone who tells you that it will take more than a week for an answer. Get to a doctor or lab that assures a prompt response.

Home Access Health Corporation manufactures the only "home" HIV test currently available. The name is somewhat misleading, because the test itself is not performed in your home, as are typical home pregnancy tests. Instead, you prick your finger for a sample of blood and mail it back to the laboratory. There the standard ELISA test is run on your blood, followed by Western blot confirmation for all HIV-positive cases. The company promises a standard turnaround time of less than one week, but an express service is available in three business days if you can't wait. The kit is available in many pharmacies without prescription or directly from the company for approximately $46. (The express kit costs $10 more.) You call an 800 phone number for results, and if you are HIV positive, an operator comes on and offers counseling. Your identity is protected by an eleven-digit number known only to you. No name or return address is needed on the enclosed mailer.

Home Access Health Corporation promises telephone counseling both before and after testing for anyone who requests it. The company even maintains a referral network by area code if you need to talk with someone in person. Many physicians oppose "home" testing because they feel that one-to-one counseling in a personal setting is crucial and not adequately provided by a voice at the end of a toll-free phone number. If "home" testing is the only way you'll agree to be tested, go for it. It is certainly far better than not being tested at all. Home Access Health Corporation can be reached at 1-800-HIV-TEST.

All these tests require the presence of HIV antibodies for a positive result. Because antibodies don't appear for up to two months after infection (occasionally as long as six months), a window period exists wherein you are highly contagious but your test is still negative. Some physicians advocate viral load measurements that detect the actual HIV virus in your blood as an earlier indication of infection. This test should be positive within one month of infection and shortens the window in which a false negative result can occur. The viral load test has significant clinical implications: Not only can it give you a true answer sooner, but it might be useful if immediate treatment is planned in an attempt to wipe out HIV before it takes hold. The downside of viral load testing is that results can take up to a week to obtain and your insurance company may not pay for it.

If you had risky sex and worry about HIV, get tested. You might already be positive. If you test negative, repeat the test in one month and again in three months. By then most men with HIV will have developed antibodies and test positive. Just to be sure, however, repeat your test in six months. (Some doctors combine viral load testing with antibody testing.)

Confidentiality in Testing

For gay men, HIV testing is not a simple matter—not only because a positive result still feels like a death sentence, but also because of the psychosocial and economic issues it raises. Most HIV-positive men can look forward to many years of good health during which their positive status should remain private. Colleagues at work, acquaintances, and anyone else you don't feel like telling should not be able to find out you're positive. How might a bank view you if you applied for a mortgage? Or a prospective employer looking to hire you away from your present job? Sure, laws protect you from this type of discrimination, but who knows the real reason behind the bank's denial or why the job offer suddenly fell apart? We have enough trouble living as gay men in our homophobic society to have issues muddied by HIV test results.

Many states, including California and Florida, allow anonymous testing. Your blood is sent to a laboratory with only a number or pseudonym to keep your identity secret.

Unfortunately, fewer states every year are allowing this type of testing. If your doctor uses a commercial lab (Smith-Klein, Quest, LabCorp, etc.) to test samples, then the results will not be confidential if your tube of blood is sent with your name on it. The lab bills your insurance company for the test unless you specify that you want to be billed directly. Although your insurance company won't know your result, it will know you were tested. If anonymity is important to you, check with your doctor, local health department, or gay community center first to find out which options are available.

Some states, including New Jersey, Colorado, and Ohio, do not allow anonymous testing. A name *must be* submitted with each test. (Table 5.1 presents a list of states that required name reporting in 1998. Note that the list is only a guide, as laws change constantly.) I know how your mind works; you're already thinking about using a pseudonym. Some states are lax in requiring proof of identity. If you go to your own doctor, forget the pseudonym. (We're not that stupid.) Choose a clinic instead. Call ahead and find out if positive identification is required.

Whether your state allows anonymous testing or not, all require health department notification of patients with AIDS. When your T-cells drop below 200 your name will be added to the list. Names, however, are supposed to be kept confidential. The information is also passed on to the Centers for Disease Control, anonymously, for epidemiological purposes.

Many people use the phrases "anonymous testing" and "confidential testing" synonymously. They are not. Anonymous testing refers to any HIV test where your identity is unknown, and you use a pseudonym, special number, or some other code to identify your tube of blood and to retrieve your result. No one will be able to find out your result unless you tell them. If you submit to confidential

101

TABLE 5.1
STATES REQUIRING NAME REPORTING OF HIV+ PATIENTS
(AS OF 1998)

ALABAMA	MISSISSIPPI	OKLAHOMA
ARKANSAS	MISSOURI	OREGON*
COLORADO	NEBRASKA	SOUTH CAROLINA
CONNECTICUT*	NEVADA	SOUTH DAKOTA
IDAHO	NEW MEXICO	TEXAS*
INDIANA	NEW YORK	UTAH
LOUISIANA	NORTH CAROLINA	WEST VIRGINIA
MICHIGAN	NORTH DAKOTA	WYOMING
MINNESOTA	OHIO	

*Requires reporting names of infected children only.

HIV testing, your name is used but your results remain confidential. Most doctors offer confidential testing because they clearly know your identity. Your HIV status will probably end up in your medical record (it's relevant), but your doctor would never divulge the result or the fact that you were tested unless you first authorized it.

In most states, HIV testing cannot be performed without your prior *written* consent. But what constitutes consent varies greatly. In some states, and New York is one, this involves your actual signature on a document specific for HIV testing. The facility is also required to provide counseling before and after testing.

It is sad that many states do not protect your anonymity or choice by mandating safeguards. Be aware that some states allow routine HIV testing in situations such as hospital admissions or as part of pre-employment physicals (as in the Job Corps). You may not even be told you were tested. Some places that require informed consent prior to HIV testing bury the actual permission for the test within a general consent for medical treatment you sign as part of any hospital admission. If it is important to you, always ask before you sign. Whenever someone sticks you for a sample of blood, ask what tests are being performed. If the technician is evasive, then ask specifically if an HIV test will be done.

New Jersey allows uninformed testing if a healthcare worker was exposed to your blood through a needle stick or other accident. (Many states have similar provisions.) A patient of mine was asleep on the operating table, and while I repaired his hernia the anesthesiologist stuck herself with a needle. A sample of my patient's blood was taken for HIV and hepatitis screening, and even I wasn't told. You can imagine my shock one week later when the man's positive test results crossed my desk. Telling him he was HIV positive when he didn't even know he had been tested was one of the hardest tasks I've ever faced as a physician.

When you apply for most insurance policies, whether life, health, or disability, prepare for routine and sometimes uninformed HIV testing. (California is the exception.) Always ask your agent if the policy requires HIV testing. Since a positive test almost universally carries a denial of insurance, know your status before you apply. When an insurance company denies coverage, it usually comes in an impersonal form letter and your HIV status may not even be listed. This is no way to find out you're positive.

There are certain instances when you cannot refuse HIV testing. Blood donations are universally screened for HIV, so if you don't want to be tested, don't give blood. The armed services require it, as does the Job Corps. Most prison inmates are tested. People applying for citizenship must be HIV tested; if positive, they will be denied citizenship. Some healthcare workers may face mandatory testing. Employers can require you to be tested as part of a pre-employment physical as long as testing is required for all employees. Individuals cannot be singled out for testing. If you have HIV, you cannot be denied a job based solely on your HIV status. (I'm sure they'll find another reason if they want to.)

There are other ways people determine your HIV status without seeing definitive test results. Do not hide your status from any physician or healthcare worker. This information is an important part of your medical record, but be careful whom you allow to see these records. If your employer needs a letter before you can return to work after illness, your HIV status does not have to be included. A simple "the patient was recently hospitalized" or "he was seen today for a routine examination" is more than enough. And don't forget that most savvy secretaries can tell that you have HIV just from a list of your medications. (Who else takes AZT?) Know who sees your insurance claims before they are sent for payment.

At the bottom of every health insurance form you sign is a statement giving the company access to your medical records should it be deemed necessary. What constitutes "necessary" is at the sole discretion of your insurance company. If you are HIV positive, this information will be forwarded as part of your record, but, fortunately, no insurance company can drop your coverage because of this. If you have HIV, do not expect your physician to hide it from your health plan or other healthcare providers. But that doesn't mean that it has to be sent to anyone else who asks for it. Most doctors use the utmost discretion when divulging patient information. You cannot forbid your doctor from including any information deemed relevant from your medical records. Your HIV status is certainly relevant, so just assume it's in your chart.

I am all for privacy as long as it doesn't interfere with your HIV treatment or other health problems. No physician can evaluate you properly for any illness unless he or she knows you're HIV positive—and not because the doctor or nurse has to be extra careful when handling your blood. Healthcare workers take universal precautions with every patient. HIV exposes you to a myriad of otherwise rare diseases that doctors may not consider unless they know your status.

Some gay men refuse HIV treatment because they don't want medication bills sent to their insurance companies for reimbursement, and the out-of-pocket costs are prohibitive. One flight attendant I treated worked a route to London, where he obtained his medications for free. When the airline stopped flying to London, his treatment stopped too. He refused to buy medicines in the United States, fearing his international flying would end if the company knew he had HIV. His logic was quietly suicidal. By the time I saw him years later his T-cells were so low and his viral load so high that he never recovered.

Besides your physician, whom you choose to tell about your HIV status is an entirely personal matter—except where a sexual partner is concerned. If you are planning to engage in high-risk sex (anal intercourse or oral sex), your partner has a right to know you are positive. Jerking off and other low-risk sexual practices are safe, and you may keep your status secret if you must. If someone chooses not to have sex with you because you are HIV positive (and that's what the Centers for Disease Control recommends), then move on. Just as you have a choice about whom you sleep with, so should your partner—and it must be an informed choice.

If you are HIV positive, you have a responsibility to protect your partners—even if they don't want it. The guy who's blowing you may beg you to come in his mouth or ask you to fuck him even though you don't have a condom. Even if you don't ejaculate, there still is a risk you can pass HIV during unprotected penetrative sex. Sure, you can oblige him, but how would you feel if he catches HIV from you? Increasingly, it's not just a moral concern; *more than half the states in the United States have already enacted laws making it a criminal offense to knowingly infect another person with HIV.*

It is never easy to find out that you are HIV positive. I always counsel patients to be careful whom they tell. Some men deal with the news by telling everyone, hoping somehow to minimize their anxiety. This is not the way to do it, and in the end you usually find that you've told people whom you shouldn't. Sure, many will want to help, but others will view it as just another bit of good dish. Friends or loved ones may have a very difficult time dealing with the fact that you're HIV positive—especially parents. Often they have a very limited understanding of HIV and are far less prepared than you to deal with the news. Of course you'll want to tell them, but it may need to be a gradual process of education and understanding.

Some men react in just the opposite manner and tell no one. This is also not the way to deal with the problem. Find someone you can trust, someone caring who will help you handle it. Don't be afraid to unburden your heart, but pick your confidants carefully.

All sexually active gay men should be tested periodically for HIV. Not only does knowing your HIV status allow you to pass the information on to others, it also has important treatment implications. Frightening is the only word for the Centers for Disease Control estimate that a quarter million people do not know they carry HIV! You may argue that your only sex is safe sex and that the test would just add an unnecessary layer of stress. If your sex is so safe, then why fret over test results? Unless you're in a genuinely monogamous relationship, all sex should be safe no matter what your partner's HIV status is *presumed* to be. (Shocking, but people do lie!) Even safe sex bears a minimal risk of transmission. If you have any STD—even if it's just a penile wart—get tested. People with one STD have a much higher risk for also having HIV.

The start of what you hope will be a lasting relationship is an ideal time for both you and your partner to be tested. Not only because you should know each other's status, but also because with time, and presumed monogamy, partners tend to relax their safe-sex vigilance. I cannot tell you how many patients I have tested, all panic stricken because they just learned that the man who's been coming in their mouth or ass is suddenly HIV positive when all along he had sworn he was negative. But before you go for testing with your new partner, examine *all* issues carefully—not just how you will deal with your own results, but how it will impact your relationship if only one of you is negative.

I also advise periodic testing for partners in monogamous relationships. An anniversary or birthday is a good time, because it becomes routine and doesn't raise suspicions of infidelity in one partner or the other. (See Chapter 10.) A small but significant number of HIV-negative men in monogamous relationships abandon safe-sex practices and become positive. This is obviously because one partner (or both) isn't really monogamous or because one didn't know he was positive when the relationship began. (Don't act so surprised!)

Treatment

He still had that boyish cast to his face, but his blue eyes looked beyond me. "Your T-cells just fell below three hundred," I said, but he made no effort to respond. I tried to catch his gaze. "It's definitely time to begin treatment."

He shook his head. "I'm still over two hundred. That's not AIDS."

"You don't want to get AIDS," I emphasized.

His jaw tightened and he leaned forward. "I feel great—not sick at all. Like this I go whole days without thinking I have HIV. If I start the medication then with every pill I swallow—five, six times a day—I'll be reminded. Reminded I've got it."

HIV treatment is one of the most rapidly changing and constantly evolving areas in medicine, but *medications should never be viewed as an alternative to safe sex.* I am appalled by men who don't seem to care that they became HIV positive because drugs will keep them healthy. As little as one year ago most physicians advised treatment only when your T-cells fell below 200. New research now supports treatment as soon as your viral load reaches 5,000 to 10,000 copies per milliliter or your CD4+ counts fall below 500. Some physicians even advocate treatment as soon as you become positive, irrespective of other parameters. But no doctor should give you medication based on an anonymous test performed outside of his or her office (from a home test kit or clinic). If this is how you found out you had HIV, prepare to be retested to document your results officially.

Many reasons support an aggressive treatment regimen. We know that as the disease enters a clinically latent phase where you feel well and the viral load in your blood may be low, virus hides in potentially great numbers in your lymph nodes. Treatment during this period kills hidden virus, reduces your viral load, and, it is hoped, decreases your ability to infect others.

Research has shown that although HIV multiplies rapidly in CD4+ cells, its genes aren't always copied correctly. An improperly copied gene translates into a potential mutation. While most mutations have no effect, some destroy the virus and others are potentially more dangerous in that they make HIV resistant to medications. If aggressive therapy thwarts viral reproduction, then it also decreases the chance of a resistant mutation developing.

You may already be infected with virus strains resistant to certain medications. One drug may kill some of your virus but allow resistant strains to multiply freely. Then you end up with an infection of more resistant virus. Doctors saw this happening frequently in the late 1980s when only AZT was available. When HIV is hit with three drugs at once, patients have a much higher chance of killing all their virus because the incidence of resistance to all three medications is much lower. Sure, some virus survives, but then your doctor will switch medications to try to wipe those out as well. Unfortunately, we are seeing strains of HIV emerge resistant to most, if not all, medications.

Once you swallow that first set of pills, you are probably committed to lifelong treatment—an emotionally and physically taxing proposition, given possible dietary restrictions, time constraints mandated by these drugs, and their side effects. Fortunately, dosing regimens are getting simpler, with the general trend being one of higher doses taken less frequently. Nevertheless, it is crucial that you adhere to your medication schedule. If you lack the resolve to stick to your regimen, you're better off doing nothing until you develop that resolve. Skipped or improperly taken medication does not kill virus and may help resistant strains multiply. By the time your doctor wonders why your T-cell counts are falling and your viral load is rising, it may be too late. You may never recover no matter what medications you try.

Although collectively called antiretroviral agents, currently three classes of approved medications are used to treat HIV: nucleoside analogs, protease inhibitors, and non-nucleoside reverse transcriptase inhibitors. A fourth group, the somewhat confusingly named nucleotide analogs, is a new class of medications. At this writing, adefovir, the first drug in this class, awaits FDA approval.

Nucleoside analogs were the original class of medications

developed to combat HIV. Zidovudine (AZT or Retrovir, as it is commonly called) was licensed first, and now there are many others. Even though AZT was shown to be active against HIV in the laboratory in 1985, it was not approved by the FDA until two years later! Nucleoside analogs resemble normal DNA building blocks. The virus mistakenly incorporates these drugs into its DNA, and the defective virus produced cannot survive. Bone marrow suppression is the most dangerous side effect produced by some of these drugs. You can become severely anemic or your white count can drop. Other nucleoside analogs cause a peripheral neuropathy—a fancy name for tingling, burning, or numbness in your hands and feet. It varies in severity and usually goes away when the medication is stopped. (See Table 5.2 for the other drugs in this class and common doses.)

Protease inhibitors have shown great promise, and drug combinations containing them dramatically improved survival rates since their introduction in the fight against HIV. Saquinavir (Invirase), in December 1995, was the first FDA-approved protease inhibitor, but others quickly followed. (See Table 5.2.) Protease inhibitors prevent T-cells from making the virus's outer protein coat. So even if the viral RNA is manufactured correctly, it has no place to go. Gastrointestinal upset, including diarrhea, nausea, and vomiting, is a common side effect of some protease inhibitors. Thankfully, doctors can prescribe other medications to combat these side effects (Imodium, Compazene, etc.), which usually lessen with time. Crixivan can cause kidney stones. Men also complain about strict dietary restrictions some of these drugs require for effective absorption. Some are taken on an empty stomach, while others need food for proper absorption into the bloodstream. It is almost as vital to know the dietary restrictions your protease inhibitor requires as it is to know the dose. Be sure to ask your doctor.

TABLE 5.2

COMMON ANTIRETROVIRAL MEDICATIONS AND
SUGGESTED DOSES

NUCLEOSIDE ANALOGS	
DRUG	**DOSAGE**
Zidovudine (AZT, Retrovir)	300 mg every 12 hours
Lamivudine (3TC, Eprivir)	150 mg every 12 hours
Stavudine (Zerit)	40 mg twice a day
Zalcitabine (ddC, Hivid)	0.75 mg every 8 hours
Didanosine (ddI, Videx)	200 mg twice a day
Combivir (a combination of 3TC and AZT)	1 tablet twice a day
Abacavir (Ziagen)	Awaiting FDA approval

PROTEASE INHIBITORS	
DRUG	**DOSAGE**
Indinavir sulfate (Crixivan)	800 mg every 8 hours
	1200 mg twice a day in trial
Nelfinavir mesylate (Viracept)	750 mg every 8 hours
Ritonavir (Norvir)	600 mg every 12 hours
Saquinavir mesylate (Invirase)	600 mg every 8 hours*
Saquinavir mesylate, Soft gel preparation (Fortovase)	1200 mg every 8 hours

*Usually taken in combination with ritonavir, and the dose for both is lowered to 400 mg twice a day.

NONNUCLEOSIDE REVERSE TRANSCRIPTASE INHIBITORS	
DRUG	**DOSAGE**
Nevirapine (Viramune)	200 mg once a day for 2 weeks, then increase to twice a day
Delavirdine mesylate (Rescriptor)	400 mg every 8 hours
Efavirenz (Sustiva, DMP266)	600 mg daily

NUCLEOTIDE ANALOGS	
DRUG	**DOSAGE**
Adefovir (Preveon)	Awaiting FDA approval

Nonnucleoside reverse transcriptase inhibitors represent a new and promising class of medications. They bind to the enzyme reverse transcriptase, which changes viral RNA into DNA, and block this crucial stage of viral reproduction. Although they work at the same step as nucleoside analogs by preventing the manufacture of viral DNA, their mechanisms of action are different. The most common side effects produced by the nonnucleoside reverse transcriptase inhibitors are allergic skin rashes and gastrointestinal upset.

By late 1998 no nucleotide analogs had been FDA approved, although the time was getting close. Like nucleoside analogs, these drugs also hamper the conversion of viral RNA to DNA, but their mechanism of action seems to be simpler. Patients treated with the drug adefovir as part of clinical trials have noted nausea, diarrhea, and liver problems as the most frequent side effects. Some men also experience kidney damage. Adefovir requires only once-a-day dosing, but it reduces body levels of an essential substance called L-carnitine, requiring you to take supplements.

All antiretroviral drugs mentioned can have severe side effects that limit their effectiveness. Fortunately, other medications treat these side effects (antidiarrheal medicines are frequently given with protease inhibitors), and dose adjustments make stopping medications rarely necessary. Your doctor won't know you're having trouble handling a medication unless you speak up. I have had patients whose viral loads soared when they stopped treatment precipitously because they couldn't take the side effects or strict dosing requirements. We know it's hard to schedule power lunches around your medications and bowel movements. Discuss your problems with your doctor so together you can adjust doses or try other medications until you strike that perfect balance between effectiveness and compatibility with your lifestyle.

Current recommendations for HIV treatment begin with a combination of multiple medications: most often *one* protease inhibitor and *two* nucleoside analogs. Again, this could have changed by the time you read this. The vast majority of men treated in this manner see a dramatic drop in their viral load to undetectable levels. Therapy is maintained until the viral load rises, a sign of emerging resistance. At this point, most physicians switch you to three different drugs. Even when all three drugs are changed, you may not respond as well as you did at first. Your virus already possesses some resistance to nucleoside analogs and protease inhibitors from exposure to your original treatment protocol. Single-drug substitutions may increase resistance and are ill advised unless done to lessen side effects or reduce dosing restrictions. Attempts to cease all antiviral treatments in patients whose viral loads have fallen to undetectable levels have been unsuccessful thus far, resulting in rising viral counts and falling T-cell levels.

Before your doctor takes out that prescription pad and scribbles illegible instructions, you must have a thorough understanding of the drugs' side effects and restrictions they place on your lifestyle. Do not allow your doctor to hand you a wad of prescriptions on your way out the door. Know what you are taking and why. If the schedule sounds intolerable or the complications too severe (especially if you already have an irritable bowel), ask about alternatives.

Know your viral load and T-cell counts. I have treated HIV-positive patients who, out of fear, refuse to know their counts. Your counts won't improve just because you don't ask, and this is not ostrich medicine where what you don't know can't hurt you. It is better to have two watchdogs (you and your doctor) guarding your health. If your doctor won't answer questions or address your concerns, find one who will!

Prophylaxis

The relatively new treatment strategy of HIV prophylaxis involves taking drugs to try to prevent infection in one of two circumstances: after unprotected sex with a suspected positive partner, or immediately upon finding out you're HIV positive. There is no medical evidence *yet* proving that infection can be aborted by prophylactic treatment in either case. So far our best evidence that this may work comes from healthcare workers stuck with needles from HIV-positive patients; when aggressively treated with antiretroviral medications, they may not become HIV positive. Research is ongoing to determine if this type of treatment is beneficial for all people (and we hope it is). For now, many physicians recommend three-drug therapy for four to six weeks after unprotected anal sex with a known HIV-positive partner. It must begin within twenty-four hours of exposure. If you are still HIV negative at the end of treatment, most doctors advise stopping medications and repeating your HIV test regularly to see if you become positive. *Prophylactic therapy must not be viewed as an alternative to safe sex!*

We still don't know whether patients who are placed on therapy immediately upon becoming HIV positive need to be treated for life. Some researchers believe that hitting the virus hard and fast can eliminate it from your system. Time will tell if this is the case.

Related Treatment

The greatest threat from HIV is its progressive destruction of your natural immunity, which allows cancers and opportunistic infections (those that normally wouldn't be able to harm you) to take hold. Not only have great strides been made in attacking the virus itself, advances also have occurred in treating other diseases associated with HIV. It is common for men with HIV to take medications that prevent opportunistic infections. Table 5.3 presents a list of the most common drugs used. Numerous other medications are prescribed as needed to combat other infections. They are beyond the scope of this chapter.

In addition to the prophylactic drugs already mentioned, you should be vaccinated against the following common diseases: diphtheria and tetanus; mumps, measles, and rubella; influenza (repeated annually); pneumococcus; and hepatitis A and B. Immunizations containing live virus or bacteria are *not* given except for measles, because the risk of infection is too great. Most physicians advise HIV-positive patients against travel to those Third World countries that require numerous vaccinations prior to entry.

A Look Toward the Future

A little more than a decade ago, there was no specific treatment for HIV. Now people are living longer and healthier lives thanks to so many scientific advances. Five years ago a typical HIV specialist spent most of the day in a hospital caring for desperately ill patients. Now most rarely have to hospitalize their patients. The future holds many exciting promises. In addition to numerous other medications currently in various stages of development, research continues to determine how many antiviral drugs should be taken at one time—or if one combination is better than another. Physicians also want to know if beginning treatment as soon as someone becomes HIV positive can wipe out the infection.

Scientists are also evaluating different tests that will, it is hoped, determine which drugs *your* particular HIV is resistant to. This type of sensitivity test is done routinely for bacteria and helps doctors know which antibiotic to prescribe. It still cannot be done effectively for HIV. Currently when a physician prescribes medications for HIV, it takes weeks of monitoring your viral load to determine if the combination is effective or if your virus is resistant. If your viral load doesn't drop far enough, your doctor still won't know if you're resistant to just one or all of the medications. Determining drug sensitivities would help tailor treatment to each patient.

And we still hope for a vaccine that provides immunity to HIV. To date, creating this has proven an impossible task for many reasons. In most viral infections, the virus doesn't change as it moves from person to person. But HIV constantly mutates, changing its appearance. Any vaccine would have to provide immunity to all potential varieties. A vaccine that gives immunity against one type of HIV might be ineffective against the one that infects you.

The search for a vaccine is also complicated by fear that immunization might cause the disease. Even a weak strain (one that can't harm you), once injected, might mutate to a more lethal variety. Such was the case with a vaccine re-

TABLE 5.3
DRUGS USED TO PREVENT OPPORTUNISTIC INFECTION

DRUG	DESCRIPTION
Trimethoprim-sulfamethoxazole (Bactrim or Septra)	Used to prevent PCP pneumonia in patients with less than 200 CD4+ T-cells or with prior history of PCP pneumonia. Dose: 1 DS tablet daily. The drug is also effective in preventing toxoplasmosis in patients with CD4+ counts less than 100. If you are allergic to sulfa antibiotics, most physicians try to desensitize you before choosing an alternative drug.
Azythromycin (Zithromax)	Used to prevent mycobacterium avium infections in patients with CD4+ counts less than 75. Dose: 1200 mg one time each week. Alternative choices: clarithromycin (Biaxin) and rifabutin (Mycobutin).
Fluconazole (Diflucan)	Used to prevent cryptococcosis and candida infections (thrush) in patients with CD4+ counts less than 100 suffering from severe, recurrent episodes. Dose: 200 mg daily. Most physicians do not recommend routine candida prophylaxis and treat each episode with a short course of fluconazole because of the significant risk of resistance with

	prolonged usage. Alternative choice: itraconazole (Sporonox).
Acyclovir (Zovirax)	Used to prevent recurrent herpes outbreaks in AIDS patients with previous attacks. Dose: 800 mg per day. Again, this drug is used only in patients with severe, recurrent herpes outbreaks because doctors fear resistant herpes will develop. Alternative choices: valacyclovir (Valtrex) and famciclovir (Famvir).
Ganciclovir (Cytovene)	Used to prevent CMV (cytomegalovirus) in patients with CD4+ counts less than 50 who have antibodies to CMV or prior infection. Dose: 1000 mg three times a day.

cently tried on monkeys. All have developed AIDS from a supposedly harmless strain.

Scientists are working with many different possible types of vaccines, from just using a piece of HIV DNA, to using an inactive virus, to using dummy particles that mimic the shape of HIV. To date, no vaccine has progressed beyond early trials. More research dollars and dedicated clinicians and scientists are needed to translate our hopes for a vaccine into reality. A decade ago there was no treatment for HIV; I hope in a decade from now there will be no more HIV!

Summary

Although great strides have been made in HIV treatment, we still have a long way to go. Increasingly, the virus is becoming resistant to medications, and a good vaccine still seems a long way off.

- ◈ Get tested.
- ◈ Anytime blood is taken or you sign a medical consent, know what it's for.
- ◈ Do not hide your HIV status from any healthcare provider or sexual partner when more than masturbation is planned. Be mindful of whom else you tell.
- ◈ Consult with a specialist regarding treatment as soon as you learn you're HIV positive.
- ◈ Take your medications religiously.
- ◈ HIV medications are not an alternative to preventing infection.
- ◈ Keep informed.

CHAPTER 6

Male Genitalia—

OR HOW'S IT HANGING?

Although in his late twenties, he still had boyish good looks and the not-quite-full beard of adulthood. He had come to me for condyloma years before, unfortunately caught after one of his earliest homosexual experiences. I nursed him through his surgery and then his difficult coming out. I knew when he moved out of his house and I knew when he quit working with his father to pursue his own dreams. I picked his chart up and smiled. I enjoyed taking care of Chad.

"How's it going?" I asked when I entered the exam room.

"Terrible," he blurted out. "My penis is too small. Can you send me to one of those doctors to make it bigger?"

Although I couldn't remember exactly what he looked like, I certainly didn't think of him as small. "Let me see," I said, pointing to his pants. Definitely not small. "You're normal, Chad. Not huge, just normal."

"This is not normal. Certainly not compared to those guys in the movies. No one will go out with me."

"You can't have a relationship because guys think your penis is too small?"

"Absolutely!"

I couldn't believe this. "Has any guy told you that?"

120

"They don't have to. So either send me to someone or I'll go on my own."

Can men really think with their dicks? Who said all men are created equal? (Certainly not a gay man.) Does size matter? Just a few of the questions all men—straight or gay—ponder through the ages. We all have one, and for most of us it is our favorite toy. But what do we really know about it, and for that matter, how much do we really need to know, other than when we play with it, we are rewarded?

Your penis is an organ just like any other, but somehow you never think of it in those terms—as, say, your liver or kidneys. And your penis does not act alone. The male genital system is extremely complicated, and all parts must work in sync for you to achieve the ultimate: an orgasm.

Men love talking about their penises in often boastful (and probably exaggerated) terms, but when something does go wrong, it's frightening—often too frightening to mention it even to their doctor. Whenever a patient hems and haws, unable to ask a question, I know it has to do with his penis. The problem can be worse for gay men because we assume that any genital problem results from a sexual act, and merely mentioning it leads to forced outing. Not true. I hope these pages will clear up any misconceptions and lead to a better understanding of your body.

Anatomy and Physiology

Your genitals belong to the genitourinary system, which has two main functions: production and excretion of liquid waste (urine) and procreation. (See Figure 6.1.) The fact that procreation is a pleasurable experience is a bonus—especially when so few of us desire to procreate. For most

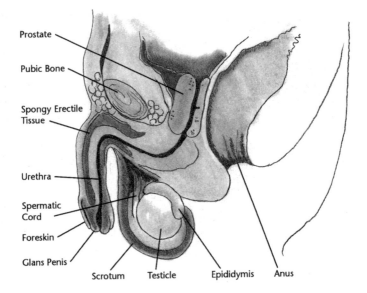

Prostate

Pubic Bone

Spongy Erectile Tissue

Urethra

Spermatic Cord

Foreskin

Glans Penis

Scrotum   Testicle   Epididymis   Anus

Figure 6.1: Normal Male Anatomy

gay men, the issues of reproduction are not paramount, and they will not be addressed in this book.

It's probably best to start with the penis, because everything else seems oddly secondary. We've all heard that size doesn't matter, yet somehow hearing it isn't enough. All men are not created equal, and if we listen to what we hear on gay sex phone lines, we'd expect the average length to be eight to ten inches with the girth of a small tree. In actuality, the average length of an erect penis is approximately six inches with a diameter of 1.5 inches. Soft, the normal range is much greater, with average being from three to six inches, and it's impossible to predict erect size from flaccid. Your penis's main functions are to conduct urine from your body and to transport semen into a woman's vagina, making size of little significance. And yes, it can be too big. The misconception that virility relates to size has screwed up so many heads and caused us to spend far too much money trying to attain the unattainable. Basically, what you have at twenty is all you're going to have.

Your penis contains three tubes of spongy erectile tissue (two on the top and one on the bottom) that fill with blood (engorge) to produce your erection. Your urethra carries urine from your bladder and runs along the undersurface of your penis. The head is referred to as the glans, and in uncircumcised men it's covered by foreskin. Nerves provide pleasurable sensations and concentrate along the top. A bridge of skin between the base of your glans and shaft is called the frenulum. Thin skin in this area brings nerves close to the surface, heightening sensation—particularly in uncircumcised men, where foreskin protects the frenulum. Circumcision is reported to decrease penile sensation because exposed skin on the glans toughens. Skin at the edge of the glans and frenulum is not perfectly smooth; little bumps (white or dark) are normal and should not be mistaken for warts or other STDs. Hair, if present at all, is found only on the base of the shaft.

Most blood flow to a flaccid penis drains directly into its veins, leaving erectile tissue empty. When blood fills erectile tissue, your penis swells, rising to an angle of 140 to 160 degrees. *Voilà,* you've got an erection. The hardness you feel comes from blood-filled spongy cylinders. As we all know, we cannot willfully cause an erection. Nerves involuntarily relax muscles in your penile artery so more blood rushes in while veins constrict to keep blood from leaving. A cock ring works because it acts like a tourniquet, helping to further constrict veins and keep blood in your penis.

Two testicles hang in your scrotal sac, which rises and falls to keep the temperature 2–4 degrees F below normal body temperature, the ideal climate for sperm production.

123

I have seen many frantic patients, their faces ashen because they've just noticed that their left testicle hangs lower than their right. Relax, that's normal, and there may even be a slight size difference between them as well. During fetal life, testicles develop within the abdominal cavity, where they remain until approximately one month before birth. Then they descend via the inguinal canal into the scrotum. If this passageway does not close off completely, you have a hole and an inguinal hernia results. Occasionally, one or both testicles fail to descend or only partially descend into the scrotum (resulting in an undescended testicle). The testicle is often abnormal and may not function. Surgery brings the testicle down and fixes it into the scrotum. (See Chapter 8.)

Testicular size varies greatly and does not correlate with general body proportions (big men don't necessarily clang when they walk), nor does it correlate with virility or fertility. (Big ones can still shoot blanks, while small ones can do fine!) Most are about the size of a walnut.

Besides producing sperm, testicles also manufacture testosterone (the male hormone). Testosterone produces secondary sex characteristics, including male hair patterns (facial hair, crab path from navel to pubis, and temporal baldness), deep voice, libido, and so on. Only one testicle is necessary for adequate testosterone and sperm production, so if one is damaged or removed, most men do fine. Fertility rarely affects testosterone, so even if you're sterile, your testosterone level is usually normal.

Sperm production occurs in billions of tubes within your testicles. From there, the sperm enter the epididymis, a comma-shape structure draped over the back of each testicle, which you can easily feel. Your epididymis, though only a little more than an inch long, is actually a series of tubes that, if uncoiled, would stretch more than twenty feet! When sperm first reach your epididymis, they are immobile and incapable of fertilizing an egg. By the time they reach the end of the epididymis, about ninety days later, and enter another tube called your vas deferens, sperm have fully matured into Olympic-caliber swimmers. Your vas deferens has the diameter and consistency of a strand of al dente spaghetti and can be felt at the top of your scrotum. (See Figure 6.1.)

The vas deferens transports sperm from your epididymis to your seminal vesicles and prostate. It is cut during a vasectomy, an operation for male sterilization, so sperm cannot leave your testicle. Your seminal vesicles and prostate contribute most of the fluid for your ejaculate; thus even infertile men with low sperm counts have normal-appearing ejaculations. Seminal vesicles secrete fructose, a sugar to nourish your sperm on their journey (to the end of your condom), as well as an enzyme that clumps semen into nice globs that stick to your belly. When you wake up in a messy puddle thirty minutes later, it's because enzymes from your prostate liquefied your semen. Is this just nature's way of forcing you to reach for a towel? No, biologically semen clumps and sticks to keep it from being pulled out of a vagina by a thrusting penis. (Some men actually do that sort of thing.) Semen liquefies when it's safe for sperm to swim upstream.

Most men ejaculate a teaspoon of semen in three to seven waves. Semen has been described as tasting sweet, salty, bitter, and everything in between. One patient swore with the utmost authority that he knew if a relationship was on solid ground or headed for disaster just by how his lover's semen tasted! I have yet to find a medical study correlating taste with disease, emotional state, virility, fertility, or anything else.

Blood, when seen in ejaculate, makes most men apoplectic. Although blood occasionally signifies an infection or prostate ailment, most often it's nothing more than a tiny blood vessel that burst from the pressure of your ejaculation. If it doesn't clear up in a day or two, see a urologist to be sure that nothing serious happened.

Circumcision

Foreskin covers the glans (head) of your penis. It is actually a double-sided flap of skin that retracts off the head onto the shaft. If your foreskin cannot be retracted, a condition known as phimosis, problems arise. Foreskins vary greatly from only partially concealing the head to dangling an inch or more beyond it. Even circumcised men can look very different depending on how much foreskin was removed. I have seen patients who swear they were circumcised, but it looks like nothing was taken off. Men can urinate without retracting their foreskins, but for sex, it is usually pulled back.

You can use your foreskin for a variety of sexual activities. Frequently it is pierced, with little or no risk as long as infection doesn't occur. (See "Piercing.") Some men try to lengthen their foreskin by attaching weights or clamps to it. Although some lengthening may result, most often this toughens the skin, dulling sensation and making it difficult to retract. Some men with foreskins to be reckoned with enjoy "docking," whereby their foreskin is stretched over their partner's glans. Their penises are aligned head to head, and any pleasure may be more psychological than physical.

The undersurface of a partner's foreskin may harbor STDs that are easily transmitted during sex, particularly docking. Medical studies prove that uncircumcised men with gonorrhea or HIV are much more likely to transmit infection during unprotected sex than circumcised men. *This does not mean that sex with an uncircumcised man is unsafe.* Just be careful! Whether the guy is cut or uncut, sexual satisfaction may not be the only thing you take away from the experience!

Jews originated ritual circumcision as a sign of their covenant with God. The practice has since been adopted by many other groups, including Moslems and many Americans. Most American males are circumcised for health or cosmetic reasons soon after birth, before they leave the hospital. Circumcision is far less common in Europe, Asia, and South America.

Arguments abound both for and against routine circumcision, with personal beliefs often bordering on the fanatical. Over the years, arguments change and so do trends. Even the American Academy of Pediatrics has reversed its position several times. In 1975 the academy opposed routine circumcision, stating that there was no medical benefit to the procedure. In light of new research findings in 1989, the American Academy of Pediatrics, in an about-face, concluded that there probably was a medical benefit to newborn circumcision.

Circumcising a newborn is a very different operation from circumcising an adult—not just for the obvious size reason. In a newborn, a special clamp is placed over the head of the penis, crushing the two sides of the foreskin together. Excess skin is cut away—without anesthesia—leaving the crushed ends to heal together. No stitches are needed. Adults have a vastly increased blood supply to their penis, so the simple clamp method is inadequate. Mature nerves necessitate anesthesia. Although local anesthesia will suffice, most men ask for heavy sedation to ease their psychologic trauma, which may be worse than the pain. After the penis is numbed, foreskin is cut away, but the two ends must be sewn together. Although risks are minor, heavy bleeding can occur if sutures open. If too much foreskin is removed, an incision can tear open, resulting in significant scarring (with decreased sensation).

Sexual abstinence for three to four weeks is a must while healing occurs.

For most of us, the decision to circumcise was made by our parents and little can be done about it. Some men, feeling mutilated, have tried to have their foreskins surgically reconstructed from skin grafts. (There is no such thing as a foreskin transplant.) Results of this type of surgery are not very good—especially since it is done for cosmetic reasons only.

If you were not circumcised as a child, your option remains to have it done as an adult. Reasons for adult circumcision fall into two main categories: cosmetic and medical. Some men think a "cut" penis is prettier and may refuse to date guys who are uncut. But just as there are guys who find uncut men a turnoff, others find them a tremendous turn-on, and there are magazines, movies, and escort services that cater to guys who like foreskin. If you're thinking about circumcision for purely cosmetic reasons, think long and hard (yes, the pun was intended) before submitting to the knife. Once it's gone, it's gone, and though the risks of surgery are minimal, there are risks nonetheless. If your partner pressures you to get rid of your foreskin, maybe he's the one who should see a doctor—a psychiatrist, not a urologist. Don't do anything precipitous just because he wants you to be circumcised. Be patient and keep it very clean. Try to get him to play with it when your penis is hard and your foreskin is pulled back. Then your penis looks almost like it's been cut.

Medically speaking, repeated infections (balanitis) and phimosis are the main reasons for undergoing adult circumcision. Sweat, semen, urine, and skin secretions collect under the foreskin, providing an excellent environment for bacteria and fungus to grow. The white cheesy material (commonly referred to by the appetizing name of smegma) has a strong odor and should be cleaned off each day. To do this, gently retract your foreskin and wash around the glans with an antibacterial soap on a wet cloth. Let water soften any crusting before peeling it off or you might injure sensitive skin. If you find yourself in bed with a man who looks like potatoes could grow under his foreskin—and you still want to stay—then include a thorough cleansing as part of your foreplay. (See Chapter 11.)

Dr. Franklin Lowe, a New York City urologist, recommends three simple steps to optimal foreskin hygiene:

1. Always retract your foreskin before urinating. Otherwise urine collects under the foreskin, keeping it wet.
2. Wipe away the last drop of urine before pulling your foreskin back down. This also ensures dryness.
3. When washing, pull your foreskin back to cleanse under it. Dry your skin well before pulling it back down.

Improper hygiene (especially in diabetics) leads to infection (balanitis) with reddening and swelling of the foreskin. I saw a patient whose foreskin looked like a beet with blisters. When it first began my patient assumed the redness was an allergic reaction, so he tried a cortisone cream he found in his medicine cabinet—anything to avoid seeing a doctor. His pain and swelling increased and he refused to retract his foreskin because it hurt too much. This only worsened his problem by preventing adequate cleansing. By the time he hobbled into the emergency room, the infection had spread onto his penile shaft and scrotum. He needed an emergency circumcision. Because balanitis is most often due to candida (a type of fungus), if caught early, antifungal creams (Lotrimin or Lotrisone) and cleansing solutions work well. Antibiotics are rarely necessary.

When infection heals, scarring develops, causing shrinking and toughening of the foreskin. At first you won't notice any difference, but after repeated bouts of infection, your foreskin is no longer large or pliant enough to retract over your glans. Phimosis clearly reduces sexual sensitivity and worsens already present infection. Circumcision is the best treatment.

Occasionally a tight foreskin retracted over your glans for sex cannot be pulled back down. It acts like a tourniquet, trapping extra blood and fluids in your already swollen glans (paraphimosis). Often men put off seeing a doctor because of embarrassment until the swelling and pain become intolerable. Paraphimosis is actually an emergency, and if ignored, you are in danger of strangling the head of your penis. (Talk about a nightmare!) If faced with an early paraphimosis, squeeze the head of your penis between your hands for five minutes to force fluid out of it. This maneuver usually shrinks the glans enough so that you can safely pull the foreskin back down. (It may not sound like much fun, but it sure beats surgery.) If you don't succeed, you'll need a circumcision.

Your doctor also might advise circumcision to treat condyloma or other STDs that do not respond to conventional therapy. If you perform an STD check, don't forget to look under your foreskin.

Proponents of circumcision cite its prevention of penile cancer, a condition not found in circumcised males. Cancer phobia is no reason to be circumcised, though, because penile cancer is exceedingly rare. Improper hygiene is thought to cause this cancer, so a good daily washing is a lot better than surgery—and you get to keep your foreskin.

Piercing

Piercing, popular since ancient times, is practiced by all peoples of the world. (Just flip open *National Geographic*.) Within the gay culture, piercing became popular in the

1950s among S&M aficionados. But piercing is no longer limited to the S&M subculture; it's been adopted by gays and heterosexuals. The Gauntlet, a piercing salon with locations in San Francisco, Los Angeles, and New York, estimates that more than half of the people pierced today are straight.

Piercing attracts gay men for many reasons, the most common being aesthetics (we love our jewelry) and heightened sensation. A nipple or navel ring can look pretty and feel great, creating an entirely new range of sensations beyond what you were used to. As one of my patients explained, "Your nipple still feels the same, but now there is another layer added to it." Some guys like gentle tugging during sex, while others find that clothing brushing against their ring or bar when they walk is exciting. One man told me that he loves his Prince Albert ring because he feels it with every step he takes, which keeps him focused on his penis and the pleasure it brings.

Most piercers will pierce any area that has a flap of skin (a piece that hangs away from your body wall) but avoid going through muscle (except the tongue). After ears, the most common piercing sites used to be the three Ns: nipples, navels, and nostrils, but now tongues are even more common.

Piercing is serious, has risks, and requires a commitment to keep the area clean for many months while it heals. It should not be done on impulse. There are also areas, particularly your penis, that, once pierced, will never close just because you've changed your mind. Diabetics have a high risk for infections and should consult their physicians. HIV is not a contraindication to piercing as long as you are in good health and heal well. Keloid formers (people prone to thick scars) should be wary of piercing because a keloid can develop in a most unwanted spot.

Piercing is not regulated by government health agencies

and most often is not performed by doctors. (You need a license to cut hair but not to spear someone's dick!) If you want to be pierced, have it done by a professional. Never try it yourself or let some friend do it. Instruments must be sterile, or you will end up with a serious infection.

Anesthesia is not required if the piercing is done properly and quickly. A needle passed through your skin creates a channel, and a ring or bar keeps it open during healing. Two stages of healing can take months to complete. During the first and most critical stage when infection can set in, your tissues are open as skin grows down the tunnel from each end. Clear yellow fluid oozes out, dries, and crusts on jewelry and must be washed away to prevent infection. The Gauntlet recommends cleansing with a liquid antibacterial soap twice a day. Infection is rare and usually results from failure to follow simple hygiene guidelines. Pulling on your ring or bar during this first stage of healing can cause bleeding and tearing. Do not change your ring, either, because you may find it impossible to get another one in.

The second stage of healing begins once your skin has fully lined the tract but is still not strong enough to withstand injury. Although frequent cleansing is no longer critical, you still must avoid rough play. Larger rings and bars gradually "up-size" your tract.

In addition to decorative foreskin and scrotum piercing, skin on the shaft (frenum piercing under the frenulum) or your entire glans can be pierced. (See Figure 6.2.) *Piercing straight through your shaft is dangerous because of potential injury to large blood vessels and erectile tissue.* Before having your penis pierced, be sure your ring or bar is properly sized to comfortably accommodate your erection and yet not too large that it slides around and damages healing. Any experienced piercer will know how to do this.

A Prince Albert ring is the most common glans piercing. In it a ring is passed through your urethra and out the un-

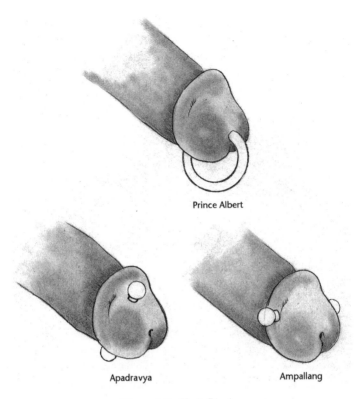

Prince Albert

Apadravya

Ampallang

Figure 6.2: Penis Piercings

dersurface of your shaft just beyond your frenulum. (See Figure 6.2.) How it got its name is cause for much speculation; some say that Queen Victoria's husband had it done to keep his foreskin retracted, as Her Majesty was offended by smegma. (I know queens with the same problem!) A pierced urethra means you'll spray, so please remember to wipe the tops of your shoes after each trip to the urinal!

The first Prince Albert I saw was huge—we're talking loose-leaf binder material—and only one thought came to mind: How ever did he get on an airplane? Not to worry.

I've been assured that the average ring will not set off most airport metal detectors. But be prepared to explain if they check you with one of the handheld models!

An ampallang and apadravya are other common penile head piercings. For an ampallang a rod is passed through your glans from side to side, missing the urethra. The apadravya spears your urethra while piercing the glans from top to bottom. (Beware of the sprinkles with this one too!) (See Figure 6.2.)

Penile piercing does not mean you have to abandon safe sexual practice. Condoms must be a little larger, and avoid ultra-sheer styles, which break easily as they slide over jewelry. Be extra sensitive to your partner's needs, because metal is clearly not as soft and pliable as your penis. Your partner may have difficulty accommodating a large ring (fold it to the side of your shaft), and it can tear his delicate anal lining. And don't forget about his mouth—no one likes chipped teeth!

If your partner did not already know you were pierced, he may be put off at the sight of your love tool impaled with a metal bar or ring. He might also worry about hurting you if he touches it. A little caring and time spent teaching him about pleasures you derive from your piercing go a long way in keeping him around for a good time. Who knows, your barbell might just tickle his fancy.

Infection is a major risk of piercing but usually can be treated with diligent hygiene. Rarely are antibiotics necessary. As with any medical problem, don't delay seeing your doctor if you think something is wrong. This is no time for embarrassment—and I guarantee you're not the first person your doctor's seen with a piercing. (He may even have one himself!) I treated a patient who waited so long that a penile abscess developed from a poorly placed direct spearing of his shaft. His infection required surgical drainage and left him with a badly misshapen tool.

Urinary tract infections (UTIs) are also more common anytime you pierce your urethra, because the metal ring or bar harbors bacteria. The major symptom of a UTI is burning with urination (dysuria). Blood also may be present. If you develop a UTI, antibiotics are necessary. If you ignore the problem, you can become quite ill.

Bleeding, a rare complication of piercing, usually stops with gentle pressure. A nasty rash frequently signifies an allergic reaction to your jewelry. Most piercers recommend surgical-grade stainless steel or titanium bars and rings. Never choose silver, because it is too reactive. And any queen knows that platinum and gold are never a problem!

If someday you need surgery, take out your body jewelry—and not because of medical homophobia. During most operations doctors use electric current to stop bleeding. There is a chance that your metal jewelry will conduct current and burn your penis, nipple, or anything else that's pierced. If your surgery is short, and you've worn the ring for a long time, removing it is not a problem. If your piercing is fresh or you don't expect to put the ring in right away, exchange it for a piece of nylon thread. (Most piercers will do this for you.) Nylon will not conduct electric current and still keep your tract open until you're ready to wear your diamonds. If you leave a tract empty, it may close.

Penile Injury

A gentle curve in an erect penis can be normal, but when severe (bent spike syndrome) it causes painful erections and prevents intercourse. Flaccid, your penis appears normal, but when hard it curves upward (occasionally downward or to the side) to as much as 90 degrees because scarring prevents erectile tissue from expanding. A hard knot of scar usually can be felt just beneath your skin. This condition,

135

known as Peyronie's disease after the French physician who discovered it, is thought to result from penile injury (bending or snapping an erect penis). If your curvature is minor and sexual function normal, leave it alone. Some physicians report successful scar softening and straightening from a variety of nonoperative therapies, including vitamin E, Potaba, nonsteroidal anti-inflammatory medications (NSAIDs), or steroid injections directly into the scar. If the problem is severe, surgery can correct the problem. A word of advice: If your penis begins to curve, see a urologist.

Priapism is an erection that just won't quit, and though it sounds like a dream come true, in actuality it is quite dangerous. The erection is not related to ongoing sexual stimulation and does not subside after ejaculation. Blood in the erectile tissue cannot get out, so your penis stays hard. Severe pain results when fresh oxygenated blood cannot enter your already too-full penis, and the penis literally suffocates.

Although priapism can happen at any age and often for no apparent reason, certain conditions are often associated with it. Most commonly they are diseases that affect blood circulation, including sickle-cell anemia or sickle-cell trait (seen mainly in blacks) and leukemia. Medications linked to priapism include pills for blood pressure control, antidepressants, and other psychoactive drugs. Illicit drugs (cocaine) and alcohol have also been associated with priapism.

A growing cause of priapism among gay men is their abuse of medications used to treat impotence. (See Chapter 7.) Viagra, the most common and available in tablet form, stimulates filling of the erectile tissue. Other similar medications are injected directly into the penis or taken in suppository form. For men with impotence they can be lifesavers; for normal guys just trying to stay harder longer they spell disaster.

Improperly used cock rings also cause priapism. Placed

around the base of the penis and scrotum to prolong erections and heighten sexual pleasure, they act like tourniquets keeping blood from leaving your penis. Choose your cock ring carefully—preferably one that opens, because it is less likely to get stuck and can be removed even if your erection doesn't subside. Cock rings also must be properly sized. Sure, a tight one creates a more pronounced bulge in your jeans, but it may not come off once you're hard. One that stays on when you're soft yet slips off or unsnaps easily when you're hard is ideal. If blood can't leave your penis, priapism or even gangrene can develop.

A friend of mine once treated an exotic dancer who worked gay bars. Realizing his tips were directly proportional to the hardness of his dick, he augmented his income by tightening a leather strap around his "talent" so he could stay hard for three to four hours. All was fine until he worked a double shift . . . and ended up in an emergency room with a purple penis.

Although priapism is a true emergency, most men delay treatment until they can't stand the pain any longer. Can you imagine explaining to some triage nurse that you've come to the hospital because your erection won't go down? But guess what—any nurse with a grain of experience has seen patients with priapism many times before and understands the pain you're in! So put on a pair of baggy shorts and hold anything you want in front of your bulge—just get to an emergency room!

Doctors treat priapism by putting a needle into the swollen penis to wash out stagnant blood. Medications that constrict arteries (epinephrine) are also injected to keep more blood from rushing in to fill the spaces. Surgery is rarely necessary.

Although doctors usually are successful in getting your erection to subside, often the damage has already been done. Unless priapism was promptly treated, chances are great that your erectile tissue was injured by the extreme pressure and lack of oxygen. Scarring occurs, leaving your once-spongy erectile tissue rigid and incapable of expansion. Impotence can be the end result.

Direct injury to your penis, whether bent, bitten, or beaten, can occur during rough sex. I have seen a Prince Albert ripped right through a man's glans, and he needed emergency surgery. Some men also try heightening sexual pleasure by passing objects into their urethra. Forget about it! This is not the way to stiffen your erection or increase pleasure. I have seen everything from pencils, pens, and swizzle sticks to glass beads and buckshot removed. Even if you put something in and were fortunate enough to get it back out, you probably tore your delicate urethra in the process. Although your urethra can heal on its own, there's always a chance you'll require surgery. Years later, long after you've forgotten any pleasure the episode brought, you might find yourself unable to urinate because a urethral stricture (blockage from scar) developed.

And what if you lose your grip and the toy passes farther up your urethra to your bladder? You will need surgery to remove it. One surgeon told me about a guy who put piano wire into his penis (maybe he wanted to hear music when he came), and it ended up knotted in his bladder. The surgeon couldn't get it out through a scope, and the man had to have his bladder cut open.

Skin disorders anywhere else on your body also can involve your penis. If you have psoriasis on your elbows, you can get it on your penis. But before you go down on a scaly red penis, be sure the guy doesn't have something else. Cracks in his penile skin make transmission of HIV and other STDs more likely.

Abrasions or superficial cuts are also possible—especially after oral sex or frottage (dry humping) when friction injures penile skin. Cleanse your cut or injury several times a day with a mild antibacterial soap—and leave it alone while it heals!

Phlebitis (blood clotting in veins) also can involve your penis. The condition, known as superficial thrombophlebitis of the dorsal veins, usually results from vigorous oral sex. (Try saying that with a banana in your mouth.) You feel a tender, hard red cord running along the top of your penis. Swelling is also commonly present. Fortunately, treatment is simple—aspirin, warm compresses, and rest (your dick). It usually clears in six to eight weeks.

I had been called to the emergency room to evaluate a young man complaining of a "facial abscess." All he had was a tiny zit on his forehead. I couldn't believe he had waited four hours to be seen for something as insignificant as acne, and I said as much. The guy (he was quite hunky) turned beet red and blurted out, "I'm really here because I've got welts all over my dick!"

Horror of horrors, it *is* possible to get welts (hives) on your penis. The most common cause is an allergic reaction to something you've rubbed it on. Men can be allergic to rubber condoms or spermicide placed in them. Some guys are allergic to lubricants or their additives (particularly oily hand creams). Topical anesthetics used to delay ejaculation are also frequent irritants. (See Chapter 7.) Allergies to antibiotics and other medications can cause penile hives, but usually you have them on other parts of your body as well. Some men are allergic to vaginal secretions, but we won't go there—not in this book.

Another common cause for penile swelling and welts is trauma during sex. A condom that is too tight—not necessarily because of size but because a vacuum forms near the tip—won't slide. If you feel this happening, put extra water-soluble lubricant inside your condom. Rubbing your penis too hard (whether with a hand, mouth, or anus) can cause a mild injury. Your erection doesn't go down in a uniform way and welts develop. This is not the same condition as priapism and usually subsides on its own. This was actually why the young man I saw in the ER had a swollen penis. I reassured him that, during sex, slow and easy was just as effective as bang, bang, bang. He blushed again and turned away, saying, "But I was on the bottom!"

Penile Enlargement

A true story, and happily not my patient: A young man lies on a stretcher waiting for his surgeon to finish the patient before him. The IV is already running and it won't be long before he's wheeled into the operating room. He's convinced that his six-inch penis is too small. He is too young to sign his own consent for surgery. His parents had to do it—he's only fifteen.

A surgeon friend of mine contemplated entering the field of penile enlargement and ran an ad in a New York City magazine offering free consultations. He received over 700 responses, and 90 percent of the men he evaluated had normal to large equipment! This story illustrates two of the three main issues surrounding penile enlargement surgery: The demand is monstrous, but true need is minimal. The third issue that must be examined is the extreme variability and sometimes disfiguring results these operations produce.

Although a legitimate medical condition known as micropenis attributable to low testosterone levels during fetal life exists, *you don't have it!* For most men, the notion of a small penis exists in their head and not between their legs. Sure, we may want it bigger, but when you take into consideration the risks involved, it's far better to stick with what you have.

The average erect penis really is about six inches—this is not a lie propagated by a bunch of underequipped men.

Does this mean that with only five inches you have micropenis? No way! Six inches is average, and average implies that normal-size men fall on either side of this number. The research of Dr. Albert Kinsey in the late 1940s measured penis size and found that 95 percent of men had penises between 4.9 and 7.3 inches. (How'd you have liked that job?) They considered anything below or above this length abnormal. (Still, I haven't heard anyone with eight inches complaining.) Most doctors today consider only those penises under four inches abnormally small. There are also genetic differences in penile size between races, and I know you know what I'm talking about. Anytime you measure your penis, expect extreme variability depending on where you place the ruler. Do you push into your pubic bone or rest the ruler against skin? And how hard is hard before you measure? Most doctors armed with only a tape measure can get an extra inch out of any penis—enough to allay their patients' fears.

Over the years numerous devices guaranteed to increase penile length and girth have appeared on the market. Most operate on a suction/vacuum principle, drawing more blood into the penis—sort of an overinflation. A cock ring keeps the blood in place. Although you may get a temporary increase in swelling, scientific evidence does not support any lasting effect. More important, anytime you overinflate your penis and use a cock ring, you run the risk of priapism. (And think how impressed your partner will be while he waits for you to blow up your dick!)

Surgical procedures to both lengthen and thicken the penis have recently come into vogue. *These operations are not endorsed by the American Urology Association. Never submit to this surgery for purely cosmetic reasons* (because the end result is often ugly), and you should never consider it if your penis is over four inches long.

I have witnessed countless men arriving at an ambulatory

surgery center prepared to undergo penis enlargement by a surgeon they had never met, known only from a magazine advertisement. They watched a movie about the procedure and signed a consent. Within one hour of their arrival they lay on an operating table and only then did they meet their surgeon. This is not the way to have any operation, let alone something as risky as penis enlargement.

Although penile lengthening and widening are often performed together, each procedure is entirely different. Lengthening surgery does not add new inches to your penis, it only increases the amount visible. A normal penis disappears into skin and fat in your pubic area, where ligaments anchor it to your pubic bones. You can feel these extra inches through your skin whenever you get hard. Suspensory ligaments support your penis so that it angles up when erect, but doctors cut them during lengthening surgery. Then the root of your penis falls away from your pubic bone and adds to your visible length. Sounds fine until you get an erection. Then you end up with what I call a dive-bomber dick, pointing straight down instead of up. Although it still gets hard and works fine, you need to pay more attention when guiding it into your partner. In addition to cutting ligaments, the surgery often damages nerves at the top of the penis, decreasing sensation.

Some doctors also attach a flap of skin and fat from your pubic region to the end of your penis, so your penis will hang even lower, even though its actual length isn't increased. You're left with a nasty scar quite visible beneath even the thickest pubic hair. I have even heard surgeons recommend that men hang weights from the end of their penis to stretch it. When all is said and done, most men end up with about an inch of extra visible penis for all their trouble.

Doctors thicken your penis by adding fat. Originally this was done with a sort of reverse liposuction procedure whereby fat removed from one part of the body (usually the love handles or pubic region) was injected under the penile skin. The fat grew there, but results were poor because fat can have a variable take—it can be reabsorbed in some areas while too full in others. Penile skin is thin and does not have much fat of its own, so any imperfection is readily visible. Most men who submitted to this surgery ended up with a lumpy, bumpy penis—their own version of a French tickler.

Surgeons now increase girth by adding circumferential bands of fat harvested from other areas of the body. In essence, multiple doughnuts of fat are sewn onto the shaft beneath the skin. You end up with a thicker penis and a tiny head. (Sound pretty?) When your penis hardens, you may see sunken valleys between ridges of fat. (Sound even prettier?)

Because the penile root lies beneath pubic skin and fat, some men increase their visible length just by dieting. If this doesn't work, try liposuction to remove unwanted pubic fat without damaging important suspensory ligaments. Both alternatives are safer and less disfiguring than ligament-cutting operations.

If your penis or testicles begin to shrink (frightening, isn't it?), this can be the result of decreased testosterone production. AIDS is a frequent cause of falling testosterone levels, as is steroid abuse. See your doctor for a thorough evaluation.

Summary

We certainly appreciate our penis and testicles from a physical sense, but we need to understand how they work. Problems do arise, and, fortunately, there are excellent treatments available. Many men agonize over size, and almost all think they're too small. Unfortunately, there is no good, safe way to make a penis bigger.

- Whenever you have a problem, see your doctor. Don't let embarrassment and fear delay treatment.
- Keep your foreskin clean and dry.
- If you can't retract your foreskin or bring it back down, see your doctor.
- Don't get pierced on impulse or let anyone other than a professional do it.
- Don't take anti-impotence medications unless you really need them.
- Don't undergo penis-enlargement surgery simply for cosmetic reasons.

CHAPTER 7

Sexual Dysfunction:

IMPOTENCE, PREMATURE EJACULATION,

AND NO EJACULATION—OR WHAT ELSE

CAN GO WRONG?

They had been together for close to thirty years, and soon it would be over. Fred, the younger of the two and muscular even into his sixties, was now little more than skin covering bones. His wig lay in his lap like a little dog. He saw me staring at it. "I can put this on if it bothers you," he said.

I smiled. "Whatever makes you comfortable."

"To tell you the truth, nothing makes me comfortable these days."

"If there's anything I can do . . ." My voice trailed off.

"There is something." He reached for his partner Harry's hand and held it tight. "We haven't been intimate for a long time, what with the treatments and all. Harry says it's not important, but it is. I tried the other night." Harry started to say something, but Fred cut him off. "You don't know everything! I wanted to see if it would get hard again."

"And?" I asked.

"Nothing."

"That's probably from the radiation destroying your nerves," I said, sounding too clinical when my heart was aching.

"We don't have much time together. And I want to be intimate again. I love him. It's important to me. Important to us. Can you help us?"

145

Most if not all men experience sexual dysfunction at some point in their lives. Whether it is that first encounter when you shot your load at the first touch of his hand or the night you couldn't get it up no matter how hard you tried, it's going to happen. Isolated episodes are nothing to worry about: They're normal. Sexual dysfunction becomes a problem when it is the rule, not the exception. The problem facing men is that we've been taught that sexual dysfunction is in our head (the one above our neck), and like all psychological illnesses, we find it profoundly embarrassing. It becomes even more of a problem for gay men who may have been taught that the very nature of their sexuality is a psychological disorder.

Researchers estimate that over 30 million men in this country are impotent and approximately another third suffer from premature ejaculation. And these figures may underestimate the true magnitude of the situation, because less than 10 percent of impotent men seek treatment.

If there's a problem, why won't we speak up? For men in general, sexual dysfunction hits us at the root of our manhood. If we can't perform, we're not true men. For gay men anxiety heightens even more. If our sexuality is an aberration, then what right do we have to ask for help when it doesn't work? Homophobic feelings are compounded by our fantasy image of the ideal gay male: pumped-up pecs, washboard abs, silky hair, chiseled face, huge cock that's always hard—the essence of virility. But if we're gay and impotent, then we better not speak up. Wrong!

Over the years doctors have made great strides in treating male sexual dysfunction. First and foremost, we've learned that over 80 percent of impotence in men over fifty results from a *physiological,* not a psychological, abnormality—most commonly caused by poor blood flow into the penis. This is a highly correctable problem.

We can break down sexual function into three areas: erection, ejaculation, and orgasm. Although these three areas are intimately related, they are not inseparable. They result from completely different physiological responses, and as such each can exist independently of the others. While it's difficult to imagine, you can have an orgasm without an erection or ejaculation, ejaculation without an orgasm or erection, and an erection without ejaculation or an orgasm—did I cover all the possibilities? Sexual dysfunction becomes easier to treat because each factor does not depend on the others. So if you're having a problem, talk to your doctor. Don't be embarrassed. It's your right to enjoy your sexuality.

Impotence

Impotence encompasses both a failure to ejaculate or attain an erection. It affects only 5 percent of men in their forties but rises dramatically to affect 60 percent of men in their seventies. Impotence was never discussed much in the gay community: First it was taboo for so long and then AIDS turned our attention from these other less-threatening health issues. As men live longer productive lives, impotence becomes a significant problem facing the gay community—and the magnitude of the problem will continue to grow. Men who have sex with men need a stiffer erection to penetrate a partner's anal sphincter. What might not seem a problem for a man attempting vaginal intercourse can mean impotence if he prefers anal sex.

Physiological causes of impotence can be divided into four main categories: vascular, neurological, hormonal, and drug induced. Vascular insufficiency represents the most common cause by far. When any part of the body rests, its requirements for oxygen and nutrients decline. The minute your body begins to work, whether digesting food or lifting

147

something heavy, blood flow increases dramatically to meet energy demands. If your arteries are narrowed by athero-sclerosis (hardening and blockage), they may be able to carry enough blood to meet resting requirements but not enough to allow for work. (Think of people with heart problems. They are fine at rest, but when they exert them-selves they develop chest pain—angina—because blocked arteries can't bring enough oxygen to their heart.) When your penis goes to work, it's in the form of an erection. If your arteries are blocked to any significant degree, you won't get enough blood into your erectile tissue to make it stand at attention.

Impotence related to vascular insufficiency usually results from blockage in large arteries in the abdomen and pelvis (aorta or iliac arteries), the main arteries in the penis, or their smaller tributaries. Any disease that promotes athero-sclerosis increases your risk for this form of impotence. Thus high blood pressure, diabetes, elevated cholesterol levels, and smoking are the most common culprits.

Vein abnormalities also can cause impotence. If your veins cannot constrict and keep blood from leaving erectile tissue (a condition known as leaky veins), your erection will not happen, will be soft, or will not last long enough for you to climax. Men with this problem sometimes bene-fit from cock rings, which function like tourniquets helping veins hold in blood.

Nerves to the penis are also vital in producing an erec-tion. They send impulses to the penis telling arteries to open so more blood rushes in and veins to constrict to keep the penis filled. These nerve impulses originate in either the brain or lower spinal cord, so a man paralyzed from a high spinal cord injury can still get hard. Any disease that damages nerves can cause impotence. Diabetes, spinal cord trauma, multiple sclerosis, and herniated discs are the most common. Neurological diseases affecting the brain, most notably Parkinson's disease, also can lead to impotence.

Hormonal problems are another cause of impotence, especially in HIV-positive men. If the testosterone level falls, as frequently seen with HIV, libido decreases and so does the ability to get hard. Thyroid disorders and pituitary tumors (prolactinomas) also cause impotence. Men who take steroids or estrogen (looking for that fuller figure) frequently become impotent. Fortunately, hormone levels (including testosterone) can be measured, and readily replaced with medications.

Diabetes, caused by the body's failure to produce the hormone insulin, which keeps blood sugar under control, damages both arteries and nerves. It is the commonest cause of impotence, and an estimated half of all male diabetics experience some sexual dysfunction. Unfortunately, keeping blood sugar under tight control may not protect a person from impotence.

Although I have mentioned many diseases that predispose men to impotence, please don't think that just because you have one of them you are doomed to sexual dysfunction. Being predisposed to something is not an absolute, and with adequate care you may be able to avoid any problems.

Drugs, both prescribed and abused, are also frequent causes of impotence and are responsible for almost one-fourth of all cases. The most common classes of drugs that produce impotence are antihypertensives (those used to treat high blood pressure), heart medications, psychiatric medications, tranquilizers, and depressants (narcotics, barbiturates, alcohol, cocaine, and marijuana). Drugs are a likely cause for impotence especially if the onset of your problem can be tied to the start of a new medication. (See Table 7.1 for a list of common offenders.)

TABLE 7.1
DRUGS THAT MAY CAUSE IMPOTENCE OR
EJACULATORY PROBLEMS*

Blood Pressure Medications	Diuretics	Antidepressants
H₂ blockers	Tranquilizers	Narcotics
Alcohol	Cocaine	Barbiturates
Antihistamines	Hormones	Cardiac medications

*Not all medications in each class cause impotence or failure to ejaculate. The complications often are dose related (increase with higher dosage). This list is meant only as a guide and is by no means complete.

Medically prescribed therapies also can cause impotence. Medications can be altered, but other treatments may be unavoidable or even lifesaving. Pelvic, spinal cord, and brain surgery, particularly if done to cure cancer, can result in impotence. (Radical prostate surgery and some types of colon surgery are the biggest culprits.) Cancer radiation treatments to the pelvic region (again prostate and colon cancers are common) can lead to impotence as well. If prostate cancer spreads to other parts of your body, pharmacological (Lupron) or surgical castration, both obvious causes of impotence, often is necessary to slow the disease. (See Chapter 9.) If you need pelvic surgery or radiation, be sure to ask your doctor if there is a chance you will be left impotent. When you consent to treatment, you're focusing on a bigger problem—the cancer. Once treatment ends and you're cancer free, impotence may not seem like such a trivial matter. New medications combat impotence, but they don't always work.

Evaluation and Treatment

A doctor first must determine the reason for your impotence before it can be treated effectively. Although you may feel humiliated by the process, it is usually painless. I urge you to hang in there, for if a cause is found and the treatment is successful, your life will improve dramatically. Most impotence evaluations start like all other trips to the doctor: with a thorough history and physical exam. The doctor searches your history for clues to causes of your problem. (Are you depressed? Did you recently begin a new medication? Do you have blocked arteries in other parts of your body? Any neurological problems?) A physical examination provides your doctor with tangible evidence that further pinpoints the cause. (Shrunken testicles, diminished pulses, a prominent thyroid, visual disturbances, a tremor, to name just a few.)

Blood tests check various hormone levels and blood sugar. A nocturnal penile tumescence (NPT) test helps your doctor distinguish between psychological and physiological impotence. Men normally experience three to five erections each night during rapid-eye-movement (REM) sleep. Expect your NPT to be normal when psychological problems cause impotence. If, however, there is a physiological basis for your impotence, nocturnal penile erections are also diminished.

I bet you want to know how doctors measure nocturnal erections. (And, no, they don't get into bed with you!) They use a portable, take-home machine called the Rigiscan. You attach its Velcro loops to the base and tip of your penis before going to sleep. During the night the Rigiscan records your erections, which doctors later analyze for frequency, duration, and rigidity.

Measuring blood flow to your penis is another critical aspect of any impotence evaluation. A painless Doppler ultrasound machine bounces sound waves off blood coursing through your penis, providing an accurate view of blocked arteries or leaky veins. An angiogram (X ray of arteries taken after dye is injected) is rarely necessary. Nerve conduction studies provide information about nerve function but also are rarely necessary.

Although I have spent much time discussing physiological causes of impotence, I don't mean to underestimate the significance of psychological causes—particularly in younger, HIV-negative men. Don't forget that about 20 percent of all impotence results from emotional problems—and 20 percent is by no means insignificant. Any impotence evaluation must also search for psychological causes. For some gay men, issues relating to their sexuality can certainly affect sexual performance. If an HIV-positive gay man complains of impotence, most often it results from either a low testosterone level or psychological problems stemming from his illness. Young men living with HIV rarely have vascular problems. Instead, heavy-duty head trips prevent them from getting hard.

Even if the doctor corrects a physiological cause for your impotence, you may still have problems. For many men, both physiological and psychological forces working together increase sexual dysfunction. By fixing a physiological cause, your doctor can unmask a hidden psychological problem. A typical example of this situation occurs in older men in long-standing relationships. Over the years one partner may lose desire for the other and their sex life dwindles. At first he masturbates, but soon he develops difficulty with even that. Out of frustration he sees a urologist, who identifies a vascular problem and prescribes Viagra. The medication brings back the man's erections but not his desire. A similar situation occurs in HIV-positive men, who are impotent even with testosterone replacement. If you remain impotent even with proper medical treatment, see a therapist. You may need to sort through psychological problems that are evident only now.

Therapy for impotence falls under two main headings: pharmacological (drugs) or mechanical. Many medications treat impotence by increasing penile blood flow, and until recently they were administered by injection directly into your penis (don't worry, it's just a small prick) or via a suppository pushed into your urethra. Now, fortunately, the FDA has approved a pill to combat impotence. The following is a brief overview of each type of medication.

INJECTION THERAPY Exactly what it says. You inject medication directly into your penile shaft. The medication produces an erection in about ten minutes, which lasts anywhere from fifteen minutes to one hour. Three types of drugs administered in varying doses, individually or in combination, are used: prostaglandin E_1, phentolamine, and papaverine. Expect your physician to try several combinations until finding what works best for you. Most men find prostaglandin E_1 gives the best results. Besides the needle, the main drawback of injection therapy is a slight burning sensation or scarring at the site and possible priapism. Injection therapy is about 70 percent effective and may work for men with more severe problems when other medications (Viagra) fail. Once men get over their apprehension of sticking a tiny needle into their penis, they find that the treatment works well with few side effects. Some even prefer it to Viagra.

I once shared an office with a urologist and watched as men who hadn't gotten it up for years dashed home with smiles on their faces and bulging pants after their first successful injection. They couldn't wait to use what the doctor had given them!

PENILE SUPPOSITORY Alprostadil (Muse), a synthetic prostaglandin E_1, is a small pellet sold with an applicator that you pass into your urethra. Discomfort is minimal, but you must massage your urethra for approximately five to ten minutes while the medication is absorbed and your erection rises. Erections produced are weaker than those after injection therapy and may dissipate when you lie down—so stay on top. Urethral burning is the major side effect.

SILDENAFIL (VIAGRA) You've heard the jokes, now hear the truth. Viagra became the first pill approved specifically for treating impotence in April 1998. Viagra works by dilating your blood vessels and was originally tested as a heart medication. Researchers had hoped it would open blocked coronary arteries, but it failed. Don't cry for Pfizer: While Viagra did little to help men's hearts, it did plenty for their erections. The drug dilates penile arteries and increases filling of erectile tissue.

You take Viagra one to two hours before sex, but unlike injection therapy or suppositories, it usually does not produce an erection *without* sexual stimulation. In that respect, Viagra approaches a natural, physiological erection that subsides after ejaculation. Seventy to 80 percent of impotent men respond, but headache, palpitations, facial flushing, and visual disturbances (things look blue) are common side effects.

While a tremendous breakthrough in impotence treatment, Viagra is not a panacea. It can be dangerous and should be taken only if your impotence is real and under doctor's supervision. Physicians have documented dangerous interactions and even death when Viagra was taken with other medications (particularly a class of cardiac drugs called nitrates that also dilate blood vessels). (See Chapter 12.)

Viagra does not increase your sex drive, only the quality of your erections. It may help remove some psychological barriers to sex by improving your erections and lessening performance anxiety. Many men taking Viagra report a generally improved outlook and feelings of self-worth.

Yohimbine, ginseng, and gingko are all natural products available in health food stores purported to improve potency, but their effectiveness has never been proven scientifically.

If a testosterone deficiency caused your impotence, as commonly occurs in HIV-positive men, replacement therapy is available in transdermal patches (Testoderm, Androderm), which administer testosterone gradually through the skin, or via injection. The two most common injectable testosterone preparations are testosterone enanthate (Delatestryl) and testosterone cypionate (Depo-Testosterone or Virilon). Prepare for a 200 mg injection on an every-other-week basis.

There are advantages and disadvantages to each type of testosterone preparation. Gradual hormone administration provided by a patch may be more natural, but many men find its daily application too bothersome. The patch can irritate your skin and prompt stares and unwanted questions in locker rooms and bedrooms. Although injections are given with a small needle, they frighten away some men. Testosterone levels tend to be high immediately following injection and low just before the next dose.

MECHANICAL TREATMENT Except for vacuum pumps and cock rings, which draw and keep blood in the penis, the mechanical treatment of impotence is generally surgical. If leaky veins are your problem, a cock ring may work; if not, some surgical procedures occlude these veins and help keep blood in your erectile tissue. Penile prostheses are the mainstay of mechanical treatment of impotence, but they have major downsides. Your erection won't look or feel natural (or even as good as the one you get from medication). The surgical insertion of any prosthesis permanently destroys erectile tissue, making medication therapy impossible.

There are basically two types of prosthetic devices: a semirigid rod or an inflatable chamber. If you choose a rod prosthesis, the doctor places one in the upper spongy erectile chambers on each side of your shaft. Your penis is stretched over the rods, which provide enough rigidity for penetration. I know what you're thinking; just forget about it. Rods do not affect sensation, orgasm, or ejaculation and won't lengthen your penis: They are measured to fit exactly what you already have. Rods come with varying degrees of flexibility or hinges so they can bend down along your leg when not in use. Your erection is not natural looking and most closely resembles a penis on a stretching rod.

An inflatable prosthesis works with a hydraulic pump that, when squeezed, sends water from a prefilled holding chamber into reservoirs implanted on either side of your penile shaft. Your penis goes from flaccid to hard as the need arises. Again, your erectile tissue must be hollowed out for the reservoirs, so if the prosthesis is removed, medications are not an alternative.

Which is better, flexi-rod or inflatable prosthesis? Most doctors I know say that the inflatable prosthesis is better because it can be inflated whenever you need it. One doctor told me that comparing these prosthetic devices one to the other is like comparing a Mercedes to a Yugo. "When you have an inflatable prosthesis it's like you're driving a Mercedes. There just is no comparison." Although pumps have many more mechanical parts than rods, they are surprisingly reliable. Either prosthetic must be removed if infection develops.

With the advent of excellent medications to treat impotence, a mechanical prosthesis should be reserved for patients who can't tolerate the drugs because of side effects or fear of needles, or for those few patients who don't respond. (Remember, if the pills don't work, the injections might.) Medications produce a normal-looking erection, and you can always fall back on a prosthesis as a last resort.

Abuse

With any prescription drug there is always the potential for abuse, and impotence medications are no exception. These drugs—whether in pill or injectable form—are intended for men who can't get it up, not for men who just want to keep it up for hours at a time. There are many reported cases of normal guys who gave themselves injections in search of the ultimate performance, but what they got instead was priapism! One patient I warned not to try it didn't care and said he was getting a friend to give him a shot for the White Party. "There'll be no stopping me" were his parting words as he left my office. He was right. Now he's permanently impotent.

Viagra doesn't require an injection, and abuse within the gay community has skyrocketed. So far no reported cases of priapism from Viagra have been reported, but that doesn't mean it won't happen. I've already overheard men saying "I did a Viagra," the way they talk about a hit of Ecstacy or some other designer drug. What most men don't realize before they swallow the pill is how bad the side effects can be. If Viagra is the only way you can get an erection, you're more willing to put up with the pounding headache, dizziness, blue vision, and palpitations. If you can get hard anyway, these side effects don't exactly enhance your sex drive. Viagra and poppers can also be a deadly combination. (See Chapter 11.) My advice: Don't even think about it.

Premature Ejaculation

I stepped into the exam room and a patient I hadn't seen for a couple of years leaned against the counter. His jeans were tight and his leather jacket draped over the back of my chair. He looked every bit as gorgeous as I remembered. "What brings you back?" I asked.

"My hernia's fine. It healed up great. Now I've got a different problem down there." He hesitated and I waved him on. His cheeks turned a light shade of pink. "I've got premature ejaculation."

My eyebrows arched. "How long has that been going on?"

"About three months."

"Only during sex or even with masturbation, too?"

He shrugged. "Never thought about it."

Before going any further I decided to ask the crucial question. "How long can you go before you ejaculate?"

"About an hour, hour and a half."

According to one medical definition, premature ejaculation occurs when you ejaculate before entering or just upon entering a woman's vagina. If you go by this definition, most of us have nothing to worry about. Another medical definition states that premature ejaculation occurs when you ejaculate before you desire or before your partner desires. Given this definition, most gay men have plenty to worry about. Many of us place too much emphasis on going forever before we finally come. We take drugs, use cock rings, jerk off before a date—anything to keep it up and going strong for as long as possible. Porn films intercut the same scene multiple times to make it seem that a real stud screws for hours and reinforce our false expectations. I say stop watching movies and get a date!

The average man should reach orgasm after anywhere from three to five minutes of steady intercourse. The operative word here is "minutes," not "hours." Premature ejaculation happens to all of us and, like impotence, becomes a problem only when it is the norm and not the exception. To understand premature ejaculation, you first need to understand the normal process. Ejaculation occurs in three phases: emission, closure of your bladder, and forward propulsion of semen. Emission, commonly called pre-cum, begins during sexual excitement when your prostate, seminal vesicles, and smaller accessory glands secrete fluids into your urethra. (Don't forget that pre-cum, while not rich in sperm, can still cause pregnancy and, more important, carries HIV.) Fluid seeps from your penis, it is not propelled as in ejaculation. Some men produce a lot of this fluid, while others may barely notice it at all. You have the most willful control over this phase of ejaculation and can prolong it with intermittent stimulation or rush right through to orgasm. With continued stimulation, the cycle moves beyond your willful control. Semen floods your urethra, your bladder closes off (so you don't shoot backward), and vigorous rhythmic muscular contractions shoot your load (ejaculatory reflex).

For most men, premature ejaculation has a strong psychologic component and is often variable and unpredictable. In some cases it can happen only with intercourse and not masturbation or with gay sex and not heterosexual experiences. Tackling the problem often requires examining your issues of self-worth and gratification as well as possible internalized homophobia.

Premature ejaculation was traditionally treated through a combination of sex therapy and desensitization. Desensitization works to prolong your emission phase and delay the onset of your ejaculatory reflex. It can be practiced with an understanding partner or during masturbation when you bring yourself to the brink of climax and then stop. Some men combine this with the "squeeze technique" popularized by William H. Masters and Virginia E. Johnson, who reported that squeezing the head of the penis or tightening pelvic muscles helped abort ejaculation. Repeat the process several times, gradually lengthening the interval until you allow yourself to climax. With time and practice you may desensitize your penis and achieve better control. Desensitization works in 60 to 95 percent of men, but after three years its success rate falls to only about 25 percent.

For men with mild premature ejaculation there are simpler methods of desensitization. A condom definitely dulls sensation and helps you go longer (and let's not forget the added safety benefit). Some men also use anesthetic creams to deaden sensation. Higher concentrations of these anesthetics are more effective and available only with prescription, but weaker over-the-counter preparations may be strong enough. They are marketed under a wide variety of names, including the catchy Sta-Hard and Stud 100. Read the ingredients before you try one to be sure that it doesn't contain anything that can damage latex condoms. Unfortunately, oils are frequent components. Topical anesthetics also can cause allergic reactions, so you might end up with an itchy, red penis. If you put any anesthetic on your penis and your partner sucks away, he'll end up with a numb mouth. Likewise, if you don't protect him by wearing a condom, his anal sensations will markedly diminish.

Prescription medications now effectively treat premature ejaculation without causing decreased sensation. Most are antidepressants, which, when taken in low doses, help prolong your emission phase. (They really do increase the time it takes you to come and don't just make you feel less depressed about how quick you shot your load!) The undesirable side effect (impotence) that sometimes occurs at high doses of these medications is modified by lowering the dose. Clomipramine (Anafranil), fluoxetine (Prozac), and sertraline (Zoloft) are some of the medications with proven effectiveness. But these powerful drugs have many potential side effects and should not be taken without a genuine need. (Not just because you want to pound him senseless!) Side effects are minimized when you take the drug on an as-needed basis as much as twelve to twenty-four hours before anticipated sex.

Antianxiety medications (Valium, Xanax) are also effective in delaying ejaculation—particularly if there is an associated component of performance anxiety. Talk to your urologist.

Failure to Ejaculate

For most men, failure to ejaculate and failure to achieve orgasm are synonymous. Medically speaking, however, they are two entirely separate functions that usually occur simultaneously. Thus it is possible to ejaculate without orgasm or achieve orgasm without ejaculation.

Retrograde ejaculation is the most common cause of orgasm without ejaculation. In essence, the body produces semen, but the bladder does not close off during orgasm. Semen shoots back into the bladder instead of out the penis. Although the condition obviously produces infertility, for gay men the main problem is psychological. Most of us need to fire away to feel like we've really come. Anything less threatens our feelings of virility.

Retrograde ejaculation most commonly occurs as a side effect of surgery. Men who have their prostate removed for benign disease can develop retrograde ejaculation. (See Chapter 8.) Prostate cancer surgery, which removes the entire prostate and pelvic lymph nodes, often destroys nerves that control erection and ejaculation, leaving men with either retrograde ejaculation or no ejaculation whatsoever. If faced with this type of cancer surgery (radical prostatectomy, certain colon resections, or lymph node removal), ask your surgeon about the risks. As with postsurgical impotence, the problem seems trivial until after you are cured of your cancer. Often there is no effective treatment alternative, so obtain counseling to adjust to this difficult problem.

Diseases including diabetes, multiple sclerosis, and spinal cord injury, which affect nerves, also can diminish your ability to ejaculate.

For most men, failure to ejaculate goes hand in hand with failure to achieve orgasm. Orgasm is normally followed by a refractory phase during which you cannot climax again. Refractory phases vary from minutes, to hours, to days, depending on the individual. Aging prolongs the refractory phase. (Remember those teenage days when you were a walking bundle of testosterone and there was no such thing as a refractory phase?)

Failure to climax is often rooted in deep-seated psychological problems. Some men can reach orgasm through masturbation but not with a partner; more often, they can climax only during a wet dream (nocturnal emission). Some gay men climax with women (a culturally less threatening choice) and not men. I have known guys who don't have a problem with casual sex but can't function in a relationship. Unfortunately, no medication treats this problem, and you must rely on sex therapy and counseling.

If you only have a problem climaxing with a partner and not during masturbation, the cause might be that your partner just doesn't know how to satisfy you. Both of you climb out of bed thinking you're to blame. In these situations, tell your partner what you like. We all respond differently to each type of stimulation, and you should never be embarrassed to voice your desires. You may like a gentle touch, while he likes to know there's a firm grip around his dick. Just because the old tricks that drove your last boyfriend wild don't work on your latest love (or conquest), don't think you're a poor lover. Ask if there is something else you can try. If he tells you there is, it's not a criticism, just a suggestion so you both can be fulfilled.

If you are just venturing into the gay world, your first sexual experiences may be too threatening for you to climax, which adds to your anxiety and worsens the problem. Start slow—perhaps just cuddling or undressing together without physical contact. (The old "look but don't touch.") Try masturbating side by side and gradually progress to touching and more intimate contact.

Fatigue (physical and mental), debilitating illness, and drugs are other common causes of failure to reach orgasm. Any depressant (alcohol, barbiturates, tranquilizers) or psychiatric medication can make it impossible to achieve an orgasm. All drugs that cause impotence also can prevent climax.

Remember, even though the problem may be in your head, it doesn't make it any less real. Help is out there; just ask for it. An appointment with a urologist is always a good place to start. Even if your problem turns out to be psychological, a good urologist will direct you to the appropriate therapist. Whether you choose a male or female, straight or gay urologist, be sure that you're treated in an environment free from embarrassment and homophobia. That's your right. (See Chapter 12.)

Summary

Most of us will know the embarrassment of sexual dysfunction at some point in our lives. But embarrassment should never prevent you from seeking treatment.

◆ Impotence in men over fifty usually is caused by a physiological problem.

◆ Even physiological impotence may have a psychological component.

◈ Medications are the best first-line treatment for impotence, but they may not work.

◈ Viagra is not the only drug to treat impotence, and it may not work.

◈ A penile prosthesis should be tried after medications fail.

◈ Premature ejaculation can also be treated with medication.

◈ Various medications and treatments doctors recommend can cause sexual dysfunction.

◈ Abusing medications used to treat impotence can be dangerous.

CHAPTER 8

Medical Problems of the Male Genitalia—

OR THERE'S SOMETHING WRONG

DOWN THERE!

Even before I pushed through the emergency room doors in the early-morning hours I could hear my patient begging for help. His partner paced outside the curtained cubicle, his face pale with exhaustion. I squeezed his shoulder and felt his relief.

"Thank God you're here," he said. "We're sorry to have bothered you, but Jim couldn't take it anymore."

"Don't apologize. I'm just sorry you waited so long to call."

He motioned toward the cubicle. "You know Jim. When he couldn't pee after dinner he thought he just needed to drink more. So he drank all night until he thought he'd explode."

"That's a common mistake," I said. "It only filled his bladder even more."

I asked him to wait as I slipped between the curtains. Jim lay on the stretcher, his hands clenched across his lower abdomen and his white hair matted to his forehead. He barely opened his eyes when I said hello.

I glanced at his swollen red nostrils and said, "You took some sort of decongestant tonight."

He nodded. "But what does that have to do with the fact that I can't pee?"

"Everything." I tried to soothe him as I cleansed his penis with antibacterial soap. I told him that in a minute he was going to feel *much better and that he'd even be able to go home. He looked away as I forced the catheter through his swollen prostate and a gush of urine rewarded my efforts.*

"Yes!" he cried out as his bladder deflated. He didn't talk again until over a quart of urine had spilled out. His relief made the early-morning disturbance worthwhile. Few things we do in medicine provide such instant gratification for patients and doctors alike.

Our beloved male anatomy gives us so much pleasure but can also bring us so much pain. If we live long enough, virtually every one of us will develop problems that require medical treatment. As we age, our prostate grows, weakening our stream from the fire hose of youth to the leaky faucet of old age. Many of us avoid doctors until the faucet refuses to run!

Our genitals are frequent targets of infection, both sexually transmitted or not. But as with anorectal problems, we frequently avoid doctors out of a profound sense of embarrassment and fear of outing. I assure you: No infection will ever out you. Straight men catch them too. If you choose to keep your sexuality a secret from your doctor (something I advise against), then a secret it will stay.

Genitourinary infections are always serious and can spread throughout your body if ignored. Read on. If someday you find that the words in this chapter sound all too familiar, see your doctor. Don't put it off until you wind up in a hospital.

Urethritis

Urethritis is a sexually transmitted infection in your urethra (the tube that connects your bladder to the tip of your penis) caused by many different organisms. You might notice mucus or pus dripping from your penis and burning when you urinate (dysuria). Over 4 million men develop urethritis annually, and like other sexually transmitted diseases, it makes HIV easier to transmit and to catch. Anyone with urethritis should also get tested for HIV.

In one-third of men, urethritis is caused by gonorrhea, and doctors diagnose the infection by culturing the discharge. The incubation period averages two to five days from the initial sexual encounter with an infected partner. Although a profuse green or milky infected discharge often stains your underwear, occasionally you might not notice anything at all. You can catch urethritis from your partner's anus, but it is far easier to give gonorrhea during anal sex than to catch it. If properly treated (see Chapter 3) antibiotics kill the bacteria quickly, but your discharge and dysuria linger until the inflammation resolves.

Nongonococcal urethritis (NGU) accounts for most cases of urethral infection and usually is caused by *Chlamydia trachomatis* or *Ureaplasma urealyticum,* both of which are frequently carried undetected by men. Herpes simplex and human papillomavirus are other, less common causes. (See Chapter 3.) NGU symptoms are usually milder than gonococcal urethritis (less discharge) and the incubation period is longer (one to five weeks). A doctor diagnoses NGU after examining the discharge under a microscope and seeing white blood cells without gonococcal bacteria. When minimal, you may have to "milk" your penis to produce the discharge. Because chlamydia is so difficult to culture, most doctors will treat you if they find white blood cells alone in your discharge. *Ureaplasma urealyticum* is even harder to culture than chlamydia, so again, doctors treat based on white cells and not organisms. Fortunately, antibiotic treatment for both infections is the same: 100 mg doxycycline twice a day or 500 mg tetracycline four times a day for one to two weeks.

Fellatio is another frequent cause of urethritis in men who have sex with men. Bacteria from your partner's mouth infect your urethra, causing dysuria and discharge. Penicillin or erythromycin are effective treatments.

One day many years after your urethritis has been cured and the boy who gave it to you doesn't even raise a glimmer in your eye, you may find yourself standing over a toilet unable to pee. Chances are you've developed a urethral stricture (blockage) after years of scarring. This is a frequent late complication of urethritis (twenty years is average), and you may need surgery to open it up. Men who've had urethral gonorrhea are most prone to this complication.

Epididymitis

If left untreated, urethritis can spread to your epididymis, the coiled mass of tubules draped over the back of your testicles. Infection inflames the epididymis, creating a tender, swollen mass. Your scrotum may redden and infection can even spread to the adjacent testicle. Fevers are common and may be quite high. In young men, the most common causes of epididymitis are STDs (chlamydia and gonorrhea). Although older men can catch epididymitis from STDs, bacterial causes from bladder and prostate infections are more common. Older men are also more likely to need urologic procedures (catheter insertion or prostate surgery), all of which increase their chances of epididymitis.

A urethral discharge characteristic of the inciting infection (pus for gonorrhea, clear or mucus for chlamydia) is a frequent symptom, as is painful urination. Epididymitis develops days to weeks after untreated urethritis, with many men never even knowing they had urethritis. Some men develop a more chronic infection characterized by months of dull pain or heaviness at the back of the testicles. The discharge can be so minimal that it becomes evident only after prostatic massage (rubbing your prostate through your rectum) or urethral milking.

As with urethritis, the doctor examines your discharge under a microscope and obtains cultures to help identify the offending organism. Treatment targets whatever caused the infection. If it's gonorrhea, expect a ceftriaxone injection followed by oral doxycycline. For chlamydia, tetracycline and doxycycline are both effective. In older men, bacterial causes of epididymitis are much more varied, and doctors prescribe antibiotics aimed at the specific organism.

Untreated epididymitis can spread to your testicle (orchitis) and throughout your body. Occasionally an abscess develops in your scrotum that requires surgical drainage. If you see your doctor early, oral antibiotics usually suffice. Delay, and you may need hospitalization for intravenous medication and possibly surgery.

Gay men who bike or lift weights risk developing an epididymitis from traumatic injury. Thankfully the condition is rare and treatment involves warm compresses and anti-inflammatory medication (ibuprofen or aspirin).

Prostatitis

I smiled as I walked into the exam room, but my new patient's frown only deepened.

"Something wrong?" I asked.

"Everything!"

I tried my most reassuring expression. "Can you be a little more specific?"

"I'm sick of going from doctor to doctor and no one helping." He glanced at a sheet of paper. "You're my ninth. I've tried so many different treatments that I have to make a list to keep them straight. The antibiotics work for a month or two and then it's back. I can't take the pressure in my ass anymore." His eyes moistened. "The last one told me I was crazy."

169

"No, you're not. If you'll let me, I'd like to try to help. I can't guarantee that I will, but I'll try."

He rolled onto his side, bending his knees to his chest. My finger went in and pressed against his swollen prostate. He tensed, holding back a scream. Maybe I could help.

Prostatitis is a bacterial infection of the prostate gland that can be either acute or chronic. In its acute form, prostatitis can be a severe, life-threatening infection. When chronic, it can be a nightmare, impossible to cure. Acute prostatitis often begins as a dull ache or pressure in the lower back, pelvis, or rectal area. The rapidly advancing infection causes severe pain, high fever, shaking chills, and prostate swelling. Swelling can become so severe that it blocks the urethra and prevents you from urinating.

Bacteria enter the prostate through a duct that connects it with the urethra, so any urethritis or urinary tract infection can progress to prostatitis. Passing objects into the urethra (especially unsterile toys) also can lead to severe prostatitis. Men who need catheters for urination are also at risk for prostatitis.

Treatment for acute prostatitis is urgent, and usually you are too sick to think about avoiding a doctor. The doctor performs a rectal exam and feels the inflamed prostate. Often the doctor cultures bacteria from either the urethral discharge or urine. When prostatitis is caught early, oral antibiotics may be strong enough. Severe cases require intravenous medication and hospitalization. Most doctors prescribe antibiotics called quinolones (Cipro, Floxin) or trimethoprim-sulfamethoxazole (Bactrim or Septra) for as long as one month to cure the infection and prevent chronic prostatitis. Don't be afraid to ask for pain medication. Prostatitis hurts.

Chronic prostatitis results from either a partially treated acute infection that never quite went away or from an untreated infection that was so mild you didn't even know you had it. Most men complain of dull, vague pain or pressure in their pelvis or rectum. They know something is wrong but often can't tell their doctor what or where it is. Some notice burning with urination or ejaculation. Fever is absent, and symptoms often wax and wane for no apparent reason. Doctors have difficulty diagnosing chronic prostatitis because symptoms are mild and your prostate often feels normal.

A smart physician suspects the diagnosis based on your history, but obtaining a positive bacterial culture is nearly impossible because your discharge is often minimal. You will probably be asked to bend over while your doctor vigorously massages your prostate. (Although most guys find this painful, my secretary has turned away patients who've come back for more!) Any discharge produced is cultured, but most often nothing comes out, no matter how vigorous the massage. Your doctor will then ask you to urinate into a cup in the hope that any prostatic secretion washes out in your stream. Your urine is cultured (it's normally sterile) and, with luck, a treatable infection turns up.

The same antibiotics used to treat acute prostatitis are used to treat the chronic bacterial variety—only the course is much longer. Expect to take antibiotics for twelve weeks, but even then cure rates average only 40 to 70 percent, with more than half of all men experiencing relapsing infections. Many doctors combine antibiotics with nonsteroidal anti-inflammatory medication to reduce swelling and decrease pain.

If prostatic massage turns up only white blood cells in your urine and not bacteria, you've got chronic nonbacterial prostatitis. Although no one knows which organism causes this condition, chlamydia is suspect. Most doctors try a one-month course of tetracycline or doxycycline in the hope of wiping out whatever is causing your misery. Don't expect much; failure rates are even higher than those seen in chronic bacterial prostatitis.

You've probably heard locker-room talk that prostatitis occurs because you don't come enough. Dr. Franklin Lowe, a New York City urologist, agrees that this is one possible cause. Abstinence leads to a prostatic secretion buildup, blocking your ducts and providing a good place for bacteria to grow. He combines antibiotics with instructions to ejaculate at least every other day. (Finally a prescription that's easy to take.)

Prostate Tumors

Don't get scared. In medicine, the word "tumor" or "neoplasm" refers to *any* abnormal growth, whether it's cancerous or not. The prostate is about the size of a walnut and shaped like an inverted cylindrical heart. Your urethra travels through it just above the heart's indentation. Before puberty, your prostate is quite tiny, but it undergoes rapid growth when testosterone levels climb during adolescence. It reaches adult size by the time you are thirty. Prostate size remains relatively stable until about age fifty, when it begins to grow again as a benign adenoma. This growth in later life is also called benign prostatic hyperplasia (BPH), and it often produces difficulty urinating. This type of prostate growth is noncancerous and cannot spread or kill you.

A prostatic adenoma usually originates in the part of the prostate adjacent to your urethra. This is important. As your adenoma enlarges, it impinges on your urethra, making urination increasingly more difficult. The symptoms of BPH are listed in Table 8.1 and result from your inability to empty your bladder completely. Your bladder still feels full even after you pee, and it isn't long before you notice the urge to go again. Men wake several times during the night to urinate (nocturia) and then wait while it dribbles

TABLE 8.1
SYMPTOMS OF BENIGN PROSTATIC HYPERPLASIA

- Feeling like your bladder never fully empties
- Frequent urination of small amounts
- A slow or weak stream
- Hesitancy (it takes you a while to get it going)
- Getting up in the middle of the night to urinate (nocturia)
- Dribbling at the end of urination
- Stopping and starting of your stream
- Inability to urinate
- Urinary tract infections

out. Remember how powerful your stream was as a child, capable of arching high over your head? Then you had so little prostate impeding urine flow. Your stream weakened during adolescence as your prostate matured, and it will weaken again when BPH develops.

BPH progresses at different rates in everyone. For some it never becomes a problem, but for about one-third of men it causes significant symptoms requiring treatment. Urine can back up to your kidneys, damaging them; or your prostate completely constricts your urethra until one day you find yourself standing over a bowl, in agony, unable to pee. As scary as it sounds to have a catheter pushed down your penis, I've witnessed men begging for it, in tears because they could not urinate.

Prostatic enlargement happens gradually, and often you don't realize it until problems arise. You adjust to having to get up once during the night, then twice. So what if it takes a few seconds longer to pee or if you have to shake more to avoid embarrassing stains? Your bladder muscle strengthens to push urine through a tighter hole, and you learn to bear down with abdominal muscles, so hard that a hernia develops. Then one day you take a cold capsule or have surgery as minor as a cataract removal and suddenly you can't urinate. Many medications, including narcotics for pain and decongestants, tighten your bladder sphincter and make it harder to urinate. These drugs can tip you over the edge from being able to force urine through a tight prostate to not being able to go at all (urinary retention).

Some men develop urinary retention even without an enlarged prostate. Any surgery is a common cause of urinary retention, because narcotic pain medications tighten the bladder sphincter and abdominal muscles hurt too much for you to push out urine. Urinary retention is especially common after rectal surgery, when the area around your urethra swells and constricts flow. I tell patients after rectal surgery to avoid all narcotic pain medications (Tylenol and aspirin are fine) until they urinate. Running water helps, but getting into a warm bath is even better. It relaxes you, so stay there until you finish urinating. (Don't worry, it's sterile.) If you try to get up to use the toilet, your bladder sphincter might go back into spasm. I have heard patients in urinary retention after hemorrhoid surgery say that their overflowing bladder hurt more than the surgery.

Some men also have problems urinating when confined to bed. They need to stand to pee, and this also contributes to urinary retention. Other men drink heavily and pass out. While asleep their bladder overfills, stretching the muscle beyond its limits, and it cannot contract when they awaken.

If someday you cannot urinate, and none of your old tried-and-true remedies, such as running the water or doing multiplication tables, works, get to a doctor. Your bladder has overdistended and its stretched muscles have lost all tone. If you wait, it can overfill to the point of exploding. You'll need a catheter inserted, but you'll feel so much better for it. Most often once your bladder empties and is allowed to rest, it regains its strength. Then the catheter is removed and you can pee again. Having a catheter inserted for urinary retention does not require hospitalization, even if it needs to be left in for several days. A bag attached to your leg collects urine, and no one needs to know. It may not sound pretty, but it sure beats a hospital stay.

If you get past your first episode of urinary retention with just a temporary catheter, it may be only a matter of time until it happens again. On the other hand, if surgery or medications pushed you over the edge, you might be fine as long you never need it again.

It is always best to see your doctor before you reach the stage where you can't urinate. BPH is a gradual process: The adenoma grows over many years, giving you plenty of time to stall its progression. A urologist evaluates your prostate several ways. First and foremost comes a rectal exam, which indicates to your doctor how large your prostate is (its size may not correlate with your degree of symptoms) and if it contains any hard lumps, which may point to prostate cancer rather than BPH. Expect to urinate into a machine that measures the strength of your stream—a poor stream indicates a blocked urethra. Your doctor may finish the evaluation by doing an ultrasound of your bladder or passing a catheter into it to measure your "postvoid residual" (how much urine is left after you finish urinating). A high postvoid residual means that an enlarged prostate stopped the urine flow before your bladder emptied. If your stream is weak or your residual high, your urologist will probably recommend treatment.

Until the 1990s, the only good treatment for BPH was surgical. Now, fortunately, there are medications that improve urination and offer an effective alternative to surgery.

Medications fall into two basic classes: those that help relax muscle and open your urethra and those that actually shrink your prostate.

Medications often used to treat high blood pressure, because they relax muscle fibers lining arteries, known as alpha adrenergic antagonists (alpha blockers), belong to the first class. When the muscle fibers in arteries contract, your blood pressure rises, and when they relax, it falls. What does this have to do with your prostate? Prostate adenomas contain large amounts of muscle cells, which tighten and further constrict your urethra. An alpha blocker will relax muscle in the adenoma, and your urine flow will improve. Three alpha blockers are currently available: terazosin hydrochloride (Hytrin), doxazosin mesylate (Cardura), and tamsulosin hydrochloride (Flomax). (See Table 8.2 for dosages.) Because these drugs lower your blood pressure, doctors recommend a small dose starting at bedtime, which can be increased gradually as needed. While taking this type of medication, monitor your blood pressure to be sure it doesn't fall too low. Other side effects include dizziness (especially when you stand up suddenly) and fainting.

Once I saw a patient with bruises all over his body. Upon questioning, he told me that his morning ritual of jumping out of bed to begin each day on a note of renewed vigor was suddenly complicated by brief fainting spells. (Hence the bruises.) Clearly, the alpha blocker his urologist prescribed caused this problem, but the man refused any dose adjustment. For the first time in years he was peeing so well. In the end, he just eased his way out of bed and kept from passing out.

Benign prostatic hyperplasia will not occur without testosterone. Testosterone enters the prostate and is converted by a special enzyme called 5-alpha reductase to a more active form that stimulates prostate growth. While castration is certainly a solution, most of us would rather keep our

TABLE 8.2

MEDICATIONS TO TREAT BENIGN PROSTATIC HYPERPLASIA

ALPHA ADRENERGIC ANTAGONISTS	
MEDICATION	**DOSAGE**
Doxazosin mesylate (Cardura)	1 mg daily; increase up to 8 mg as needed
Tamsulosin hydrochloride (Flomax)	0.4 mg daily 1/2 hour after meals
Terazosin hydrochloride (Hytrin)	1 mg at bedtime; increase up to 10 mg as needed

5-ALPHA REDUCTASE INHIBITORS	
MEDICATION	**DOSAGE**
Finasteride (Proscar)	5 mg daily

testicles and deal with BPH if it becomes a problem. Fortunately, a medication called finasteride (Proscar) blocks the conversion of testosterone to its active form. (See Table 8.2.) Your prostate thinks you've been castrated, but the the rest of your body doesn't! Side effects are minimal and most notably include a decreased volume of ejaculate. Proscar works by gradually shrinking your prostate; it may take weeks to months before you see a pronounced improvement in urination. Many doctors combine an alpha-blocking medication with Proscar so that you see more immediate results.

If you notice your stream weakening or perhaps you now get up twice a night instead of once, what can you do short of going on prescription medications? Health food stores sell various plant extracts, including saw palmetto berry and *Pygeum africanum,* that help alleviate symptoms and improve urine flow.

Most physicians begin treatment for BPH with medication, either alpha blockers or 5-alpha reductase inhibitors, or a combination of both. If medications don't work or if your symptoms progress, your doctor might recommend a number of options short of actually removing your prostate.

Balloon dilatation was met with a flurry of interest when first introduced in 1984. In this procedure, either a urologist or a radiologist passes a small deflated balloon up your urethra to your prostate. When the balloon is inflated, it pushes away your enlarged prostate and stretches your narrowed urethra. Then the balloon is removed, and your stream may improve. Although the procedure is relatively simple to perform, results have not been that good and most doctors don't recommend it.

Newer and more successful therapies involve heating the prostate immediately surrounding your urethra to the point where a portion of it burns away. The heat does not penetrate more than a few millimeters from your urethra, so most of your prostate is left intact. The dead tissue falls away, creating a wider opening for urine flow. Transurethral needle ablation (TUNA) heats your prostate with radio-frequency waves transmitted through a fine needle passed down your urethra into the prostate. Lasers also have come into vogue for destroying enlarged prostate tissue. The Yag laser was one of the first employed but is now being supplanted by the Indigo laser, which heats the prostate immediately surrounding your urethra to the boiling point (212 degrees F, or 100 degrees C) in three minutes.

Although technically a surgical procedure, prostate heat ablation has many advantages over standard surgery. It can be performed with minimal anesthesia either in a urologist's office or on an outpatient basis, and blood loss is negligible. Because most of your prostate is left intact, complications such as retrograde ejaculation, incontinence, and impotence seen after standard prostate removal are much rarer.

If you have a very large prostate or fail one of the simpler ablative procedures, you'll probably need an open prostatectomy. This type of surgery has a much higher success rate for improving urination in men with large prostates. It can be accomplished either through your urethra or through a cut in your lower abdomen.

Transurethral prostatectomy (TURP) is commonly called a scraping. Your urologist passes a cystoscope down your penis to the prostate and then cuts enough of it away to open up your urethra. This surgery requires hospitalization, and bleeding can be heavy. Most men experience retrograde ejaculation as a side effect after this type of prostatectomy, but impotence and incontinence are rare.

If your prostate is very large and your surgeon does not think enough can be removed via a TURP, you'll need an open prostatectomy. Again hospitalization is required, but because your entire prostate is removed through an incision just above your pubic bone, the success rate for improving urination approaches 100 percent. However, your risks of retrograde ejaculation, incontinence, and impotence are higher than with a TURP because the surgery is more extensive.

If you have early symptoms of prostate trouble, see your urologist to be sure that you don't have cancer. If you just have BPH, consider one of the natural remedies first before progressing to prescription medications. If medications fail, prostate heat ablation can be very effective for small adenomas. If these methods don't work or if your prostate is too large, most urologists try a TURP before an open prostatectomy.

179

Prostate Cancer

Just the name is frightening. And it should be. Outside of skin cancer, this is the most common cancer in men, and almost 20 percent of us will have it at some point in our lives. For blacks, the incidence is twice as high as it is for whites. That's the bad news. The good news is that it is a relatively slow-growing cancer that takes many years before it can spread and kill you. Most men with prostate cancer die of something else long before their tumor would have killed them. Even with slow growth, however, prostate cancer is the second-leading cause of male cancer deaths (over 40,000 in 1997), but survival rates are improving through early diagnosis and better treatment. Today doctors estimate that over half of all prostate malignancies are discovered before they spread outside of the prostate. The five-year survival rate in these cases approaches 100 percent.

Most prostate cancers begin in the more peripheral regions of the gland, where smaller nodules can be felt on rectal examination. Doctors estimate that it takes fifteen years for these earliest prostate tumors to grow and spread throughout the body. As the tumor grows, it breaks through the prostate's capsule (outer wall) and invades the seminal vesicles and bladder. Finally it spreads to the pelvic lymph nodes, bones, liver, lungs, and brain.

Clearly doctors would like either to prevent prostate cancer or to diagnose it while it is still curable. As far as prevention is concerned, some evidence suggests that vitamin E supplements may help. Doctors hope to learn whether hormone therapy or 5-alpha reductase inhibitors used to treat BPH might also offer protection against cancer.

Early prostate cancer, unfortunately, produces few signs and symptoms. By the time men have symptoms of bone

180

pain or blood in their urine, it may already be too late. To diagnose prostate cancer early, doctors rely on a good rectal examination and measuring the prostate-specific antigen (PSA) level in the blood. With a rectal examination, the doctor carefully feels your prostate for any suspicious nodules. In BPH, the entire prostate tends to enlarge; malignant tumors are often solitary, small, hard lumps within the gland.

PSA, an enzyme manufactured only by prostate cells, liquefies those nice little clumps of semen after you ejaculate. Some of it spills naturally into your blood (don't worry, it won't hurt you), and a blood test can measure the level. Cancer cells generally produce much more PSA than normal cells, so blood levels rise in men with prostate cancer. Your PSA level also increases from BPH, prostatitis, or after prostate biopsy or injury. (Use your imagination.) Normal PSA levels are less than 4 nanograms per milliliter. The higher your PSA goes, the greater the likelihood that you have cancer.

Neither a rectal examination nor a PSA measurement is foolproof. Each test misses cancers in some men and wrongly predicts them in others. But together, they are our best tools for early diagnosis of prostate malignancies. *Currently the American Cancer Society recommends a yearly PSA and rectal examination in all men over age fifty.* For blacks and men with a close family history of prostate cancer (fathers, brothers, or grandfathers with the disease), the age for yearly screening is pushed back to forty. Because the disease spreads so slowly, screening past the age of seventy is not recommended. (In other words, if you're over seventy and develop prostate cancer, you'll probably die from some other cause.)

If a doctor suspects a prostate tumor, you'll need a transrectal ultrasound and needle biopsy. A small lubricated probe inserted (painlessly) into your rectum bounces sound waves into your prostate, making even the tiniest nodules visible. The ultrasound picture guides the doctor's insertion of a very skinny needle through your rectum into your prostate to obtain a cell sample. These cells are then studied under a microscope to determine if indeed you have prostate cancer. Ultrasound guided biopsy does not require hospitalization or anesthesia and often can be performed right in the doctor's office. If the initial attempt failed to diagnose a cancer, a still-suspicious doctor might advise an additional biopsy, because 15 percent of the time the first biopsy is negative while the second one finds cancer. Early detection means the difference between a cure and certain death, so please don't refuse a biopsy if your doctor advises.

Prostate cancer does not mean the end of the world. When it is caught early, before it has spread, it is a curable disease. Even when prostate cancer has spread, excellent treatment options can guarantee you a long life. Doctors usually propose one of three different treatments for men with prostate cancer: surgery, radiation therapy, or doing nothing at all. I'm sure your eyebrows rose at the prospect of doing nothing: How can a doctor just leave you with a cancer? The answer is simple. If your probable survival even without prostate cancer is limited (less than 10 years), no treatment may be the best treatment of all.

Radical surgery and radiation therapy are the best ways to cure prostate cancer. A radical prostatectomy removes the entire gland and surrounding lymph nodes. Nerves that control your erection run nearby. In the past they were routinely cut out along with the tumor, leaving many men impotent. Now surgeons try to save at least some of these nerves, so the chance of impotence for men under sixty is less than 50 percent. Impotence after prostate surgery can be cured with medications or a penile prosthesis. (See Chapter 7.) Other frequent, troubling side effects of the surgery include no ejaculation (you still have an orgasm, but nothing shoots out) and urinary incontinence (failure to control your urine). Many men note mild stress incontinence (they dribble urine if they sneeze, cough, or bear down on abdominal muscles), but sanitary pads usually handle this problem. Complete incontinence is a significant problem for less than 5 percent of men after radical prostatectomy. Some may need surgery to correct it, while others wear a bag to catch leaking urine. Many years after any type of prostate surgery men may develop a bladder stricture from scarring, which blocks urine flow. Often a surgeon will dilate the stricture, which relieves the problem. Occasionally, further surgery is necessary. All in all, the prognosis for fifteen-year survival after radical prostatectomy for a localized cancer (one that didn't spread) approaches 90 percent.

Radiation is another excellent treatment alternative for prostate cancer that has not spread, and its fifteen-year survival rates reach 85 percent. Radiation therapy, spaced over seven weeks, kills cancer cells and can damage other structures in the beam's path. Accordingly, even though the treatment itself is painless, nerves controlling erections can be destroyed, leaving 50 percent of men impotent. Because intestines, bladder, and rectum are often in the path of the radiation beam, patients undergoing radiation treatment can expect some indigestion with crampy pain, bowel irregularity, rectal bleeding, and painful, frequent bloody urination. Sounds horrible, I know, but often these symptoms are mild, easily managed with medication, and they usually resolve or lessen once your treatment ends. Less than 5 percent of men experience urinary incontinence after radiation therapy.

Which is better, radiation or surgery? Radiation therapy has the significant advantage of not requiring surgery with all its attendant risks (bleeding, prolonged hospitalization, etc.), but it does require a significant time commitment.

Although survival rates are fairly similar for early prostate cancer whether it's treated surgically or with radiation, most doctors believe that in a relatively healthy man with a life expectancy of greater than ten years, a radical prostatectomy is preferred. Surgical survival rates surpass radiation therapy as a man lives longer than ten years after treatment.

If faced with the frightening prospect of metastatic prostate cancer (cancer that has spread to other parts of your body), try to remember that all is not lost. Although prostate cancer is relatively resistant to most common chemotherapy drugs, it is very sensitive to hormone therapy. Prostate cells depend on testosterone to grow normally, and so do prostate cancer cells. Even if cancer has spread, anything that decreases testosterone levels impedes its growth. Castration is the obvious best method for lowering testosterone levels, and it is a safe and risk-free operation. Fake testicles inserted into the scrotum feel like normal balls. (If this is important to you, ask your doctor before the surgery.) For most men, a surgical castration is too disturbing. Instead they opt for medical castration, which is accomplished with various drugs.

The most common form of pharmacological castration is a class of drugs called luteinizing hormone-releasing hormone agonists (LHRH), a fancy name for something that basically tells your testicles not to make testosterone. Leuprolide acetate (Lupron) or goserelin acetate (Zoladex) are administered via injection once a month. Side effects are similar to castration—loss of libido and impotence. Some men develop hot flashes and other menopause-type symptoms. Initially, these medications can cause *increased* testosterone levels with worsening of the cancer. To combat this, a doctor may add another antitestosterone medication (flutamide [Eulexin], nilutamide [Nilandron], or bicalutamide [Casodex]) for the first week or two of therapy.

After medical or surgical castration, most men go into

remission with either a regression of their cancer and/or a slowing of its progression. Many times they can look forward to several years of good life. Doctors are also testing cancer cells, looking for factors that predict whether the tumor will grow quickly or not. More aggressive treatment might be indicated for men with fast-growing tumors, whereas doctors would be more inclined to just watch slow tumors. If men develop urinary obstruction from prostate cancer, many doctors combine hormone therapy with a TURP (scraping) to open the urethra. Radiation therapy is also beneficial when cancer has spread to bones and other organs.

Scrotum and Testicles

Now for the second most favorite part of most men's anatomy. You may think of your scrotum as just a sac of wrinkled, thin skin, but it performs the complex function of regulating testicular temperature. Just as women are taught to examine their breasts, men must learn the importance of regular scrotal checks—especially young men, who are at greatest risk for testicular cancers. And your testicles aren't the only structures your scrotum holds. It also contains your spermatic cord with its many vessels that bring blood to and from your testicles. Your epididymis, which is draped over the back of each testicle, is another important part of your scrotum. (See Chapter 6.)

Because your scrotum rises and falls to keep your testicles at exactly the right temperature, examine it when it is fully extended so you can feel its entire contents. When pulled up tight, your epididymis and spermatic cord may be out of reach. You may find it easier to examine your partner and for him to examine you—just don't incorporate the exam into foreplay, because sexual stimulation draws the scrotum up, limiting your ability to feel individual structures. Some doctors recommend examining your scrotum in a shower or bath, because hot water makes it as floppy as possible. While that is certainly an option, it is difficult to see skin properly under water, and a visual inspection is an integral part of any examination.

Begin your examination with a visual inspection in a well-lighted setting. Carefully spread your pubic hair so that you can see all areas. Some men find shaving the hair from their scrotum a pleasurable experience as the razor glides over sensitive skin. Just beware of nicks, which can become infected, or ingrown hair follicles. Any swelling or redness after shaving needs warm compresses, frequent cleansing with antibacterial soap, and possibly even antibiotics. As with any infection, don't wait too long to see a physician.

When examining your scrotum, look for any *new* lumps, bumps, or blemishes. Any skin disease you have elsewhere (psoriasis, fungal infections, moles, etc.) can spread to your scrotum. Because your scrotum is not normally smooth, it is important that you examine any skin abnormality for change. A mole that you have had for years is not a problem unless it starts growing or darkens. Beware of any STD—particularly warts and herpes, which can infect your scrotum and are easily overlooked. Warts are often mistaken for skin tags, especially if you don't have them anywhere else. If in doubt, have your doctor check you out! If you're wondering about a little bump that grew after shaving and probably results from irritation, stop shaving for a month or two and see if it shrinks or disappears. You may get your answer without a trip to your doctor.

Once your visual inspection is complete, move on to a manual examination. Gently hold your testicle (first one, then the other) between thumb and forefinger and work your fingers methodically over the surface from top to bottom, then front to back. (See Figure 8.1.) Your testicle

To examine your testicle, gently hold it between your thumb and forefinger and carefully work your fingers over the surface top to bottom and front to back.

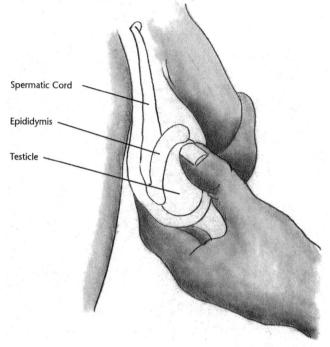

Spermatic Cord

Epididymis

Testicle

Figure 8.1: Testicular Examination

should have a uniform consistency. Any hard lumps or irregularities, no matter the size, need to be shown to a doctor. Don't be afraid of pushing one testicle across to the other side. The two halves of your scrotum are separated by a membrane. Some men worry that they will push their testicle up and out of their scrotum, where it will get stuck in their inguinal canal. Impossible. Your testicle rises and falls with your spermatic cord, and as long as your testicle descended properly, it will never leave your scrotum.

Testicular lumps might mean cancer and should never

be ignored. Testicular cancer is the most common cancer in men between the ages of twenty and thirty-four, and it affects whites more often than blacks. Because it attacks men at an age when most never think of their own mortality and the possibility of any cancer seems remote, the diagnosis is often delayed until the tumor is too large to ignore and the cancer has already spread. If you had an undescended testicle, you are almost fifteen times more likely to develop a cancer in that testicle even if it was surgically brought down into your scrotum. If you have some vague memories of some type of testicle surgery, find out what was done. (It might have been a hernia operation or hydrocele repair.) You need to know whether you had an undescended testicle so that you can be extra vigilant in guarding against cancer. Besides cosmetic improvement, the main advantage of an orchiopexy (sewing an undescended testicle into the scrotum) is that it places the abnormal testicle in a location where it can be examined easily.

For most men, a painless lump is the first sign of testicular cancer. Although pain, if present, usually signifies an infection, it can also mean cancer. Occasionally young men are treated with antibiotics for months because their doctor erroneously suspects chronic epididymitis. I know of a patient who, fed up with his persistent pain despite antibiotics, stopped returning to his urologist for further evaluations. The next time he saw a doctor was because he coughed up blood—from cancer that had spread to his lungs.

If your doctor confirms the presence of a lump in your testicle, you will need a sonogram. This painless examination utilizes sound waves to paint a picture of your testicle. Tumors differ in consistency from normal tissue, and the sonogram picks up this difference. If the sonogram confirms a tumor, prepare for surgery. To prevent the spread of cancer, your doctor will remove your testicle through an incision in your groin rather than your scrotum. A prosthetic testicle can be inserted in its place. A seminoma is the most common type of testicular cancer, and it is highly sensitive to radiation and chemotherapy. Radiation treatments often are used after surgery to improve cure rates to close to 95 percent.

After you've examined your testicle, move toward the back and feel your epididymis, which drapes over the top and back of your testicle like a comma. It is even more sensitive than your testicle, so be extra gentle. Be sure it's free of lumps or undue tenderness. Small lumps are usually fluid-filled cysts, not tumors. Milky white fluid indicates a spermatocele (a cyst containing sperm). Most cysts are pea size, but occasionally they can grow large. No treatment is necessary unless they cause pain, and in that case the doctor can remove the cyst through a tiny incision in your scrotum.

At the top of your scrotum, feel your spermatic cord. It should be no thicker than your index finger, and you can recognize it by the hard tube running within it—your vas deferens. The spermatic cord exits the top of your scrotum and runs in your inguinal canal for several inches before diving through the muscles of your abdominal wall.

An enlarged spermatic cord can signify a varicocele, which means varicose veins of your cord. (See Figure 8.2.) A varicocele often feels like a bag of worms (medical imagery, not mine) that you can squish between your fingers. When you stand, these veins are sometimes visible in a tangle just beneath your skin surface. Varicoceles are more common on the left side but may affect both sides. They raise the temperature inside your scrotum by keeping extra blood around the testicle. With time and increased temperatures, the testicle will atrophy (shrink) and become infertile. For gay men this is usually of little consequence. Have

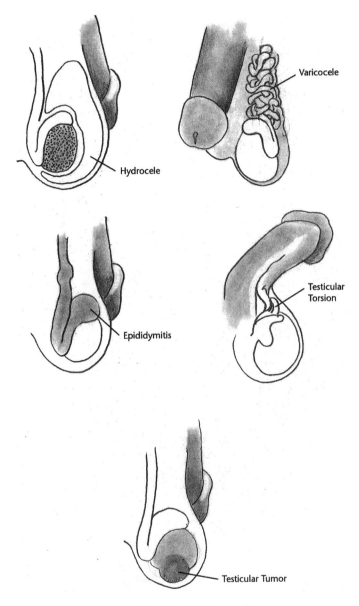

Figure 8.2: Testicle Abnormalities

your varicocele fixed if you have symptoms of back pain and heaviness in your scrotum.

Testicular torsion occurs when a testicle twists around on your spermatic cord. You have every right to wince, because this is an extremely painful (emphasis on extremely) situation. When the spermatic cord twists, the blood flow to your testicle cuts off and the testicle strangles. Onset of severe pain is sudden, and most men begin to vomit. Your twisted testicle is often higher in your scrotum than normal, and pain makes it impossible to touch. You need emergency surgery to untwist the testicle. Delay, and your doctor will probably have to remove it. Although testicular torsion can strike at any age, it is far more common in men between puberty and their mid-twenties.

An enlarging testicle does not necessarily mean cancer. A hydrocele is a painless collection of fluid around a testicle; it may be small or may reach enormous proportions. (We're talking grapefruits.) (See Figure 8.2.) Unlike a tumor, a hydrocele is uniform in size and consistency. (Think of your testicle lying inside a water balloon.) An easy trick to use to diagnose a hydrocele yourself is to shine a flashlight against your scrotum while in a darkened room. The fluid in a hydrocele lights up like a globe, but tumors or normal testicles won't transmit light. Hydroceles are not dangerous and need to be surgically removed only in those instances when their size becomes a problem. Except for pressure from fluid buildup, they are usually painless.

An inguinal hernia is a hole in the abdominal muscles through which abdominal organs protrude. The hole usually lies somewhere along the path the testicle traveled on its way into your scrotum before birth. If ignored, a hernia can grow so large that it ends up in your scrotum. Hernias should be surgically repaired, because abdominal organs can get stuck in them (incarcerate) and even strangulate and die. Then what would have been a simple outpatient surgery becomes a life-or-death emergency requiring hospitalization.

I once treated a man who had a huge hernia (the size of a small melon) in his left scrotum. Although he had ignored it for years, for some reason he suddenly wanted it repaired. (Summer was coming and maybe he wanted to wear shorts for the first time in years.) His hernia was so large that I could not feel his testicle, which had been undescended and brought into his scrotum when he was five. During surgery, I pushed his hernia back into his abdomen, and then I could feel his testicle. Although shrunken and probably nonfunctional, it had a tiny rock-hard nodule in it. I took a biopsy and it turned out he had a seminoma. I removed his entire testicle and spermatic cord. Fortunately, the tumor was found early and had not had a chance to spread. If he had not suddenly wanted his hernia repaired, his testicle never could have been felt, and the tumor undoubtedly would have spread.

Women have been conditioned to go to their gynecologist for routine checkups, but men avoid urologists. I hope you've learned from these pages how complex our male anatomy really is. We take it for granted when instead we need to afford ourselves the same care women have come to expect.

Summary

It isn't enough to go to a urologist only when something is wrong. Testicular tumors strike young men who never consider their own mortality. As we age, our prostates become potentially lethal time bombs, and men over fifty must be checked regularly. Don't think of a trip to a urologist as an assault on your manhood. They're there to protect what you've got. And if you're too embarrassed to drop your pants, remember: They've seen it all before.

- ◈ Your doctor should examine any urethral discharge.
- ◈ If you have urethritis, get HIV-tested.
- ◈ Chronic prostatitis is very difficult to cure. Don't give up.
- ◈ All men between fifty and seventy need yearly prostate examinations and PSA levels to screen for prostate cancer.
- ◈ If you have prostate cancer, discuss treatment options with your doctor to determine which is best for you.
- ◈ Get in the habit of regularly examining your testicles.
- ◈ Show any scrotal lumps to your doctor.
- ◈ Don't ignore genital pain.

CHAPTER **9**

Oral Sex—

OR PLEASE TELL ME IT'S SAFE

I listened intently. *My patient was nervous, his embarrassment overcome only by his fear of not knowing for sure.*

He wiped his sweaty palms against his shirt. "The guy told me it was safe. I'd never done it before."

"Done what?" I asked. I had long ago learned never to assume anything.

"You know, oral sex."

Still not assuming, I asked, "What kind of oral sex?"

He hesitated before adding "With water."

"Water, as in water sports?"

His eyes widened and words poured out. "He wanted to pee in my mouth. First I did it to him and then he wanted to do it to me. I'd never done that before. He said it was safe—a lot safer than coming."

"And now you're worried about it."

He nodded. "It's safe, right?"

For gay men, oral sex is one of our most intimate sexual acts. And after mutual masturbation, fellatio might be an adolescent's next tentative foray into the world of gay sex—even before that first deep kiss.

But is it safe? Herein lies one of the most controversial

194

issues in gay sex; a topic debated, expounded upon, forbidden, and embraced (and often all on the same day) by homosexuals and heterosexuals alike. The Centers for Disease Control, playing it very safe, goes so far as to say that condoms should be used for *all* oral sex. But fellatio runs the gamut from merely taking a penis into your mouth to swallowing your partner's semen (or urine)—and everything in between. By definition, it also includes rimming (oral-anal sex) and even kissing. Your risk for catching HIV and many other sexually transmitted diseases depends on where along the spectrum your proclivities lie.

Fellatio

I am not going to teach you how to give a blow job. You're probably already a pro. But I will give you a few pointers. Before you take your partner into your mouth, use your eyes to be sure he's clean. If he is uncircumcised, pull back his foreskin and take a good look. Wipe away any smegma, but don't embarrass him. Disguise hygiene as part of your foreplay.

The main problem most men face during oral sex is that darn "gag" reflex. As my grandmother used to say, "Your appetite is bigger than your stomach." The same holds true for gay men and oral sex. Our mouths are only so big, while our appetites are huge—the bigger the penis, the more the thrill. Just as we want that extra piece of chocolate cake even though we're stuffed to the gills, we also want that extra inch even though he's already banging our tonsils.

Your gag reflex is not merely a nuisance. It is a highly protective neurological and muscular chain of events that prevents food from getting trapped in your trachea (windpipe) or lungs. There are two passages at the back of your mouth: your trachea, which carries air from the nose and mouth to your lungs, and your esophagus, which transports food to your stomach. When you swallow, your trachea closes, so food enters only your esophagus. This makes it impossible to drink and breathe at the same time. If your trachea isn't closed and food hits the back of your throat, your brain immediately sends a signal to muscles in your chest and mouth, forcing you to gag. This propels food out of the way. People who lose their gag reflex (as happens to some stroke victims) often develop terrible pneumonia when food and saliva travel into their lungs (aspiration).

Gagging clearly can be suppressed—just look at sword swallowers. Some of it is in our heads, and relaxing during oral sex may go a long way to minimizing your urge to gag. If the very thought of oral sex is a turnoff, but you want to try because it is important to your partner, coat his penis with something delicious to eliminate any musty odors or taste. Some men prefer a bit of jelly or honey with their penis, while fancy queens insist on caviar. Avoid foods containing oils and fat when using a condom.

If your partner is large, you can keep from gagging by taking only part of it into your mouth. Stimulate the base of his shaft with your free hand. His pleasurable sensations centered mainly about his glans are probably not minimized and may even be heightened because your tongue and lips stimulate this area better. Some men decrease gagging by breathing in through their nose while they travel downward on their partner's shaft. Others find just the opposite is true, that holding their breath is the answer.

If your partner is very thick as well as long, he will hit more of the back of your throat and stimulate gagging. Sword swallowers keep from vomiting and impaling themselves on their spears by adjusting the angle of their neck so nothing touches the back of their throat. (Unlike many gay men, they also avoid thick swords.) Learn from these circus performers by angling your head back to change the angle of your partner's penetration, so his penis is better aligned with your esophagus and not the back of your throat.

Many mouthwashes or lozenges marketed as sore throat remedies contain topical anesthetics that deaden nerves at the back of your throat. If you really want to go down on "Mr. Big" but can't keep from gagging, try one of these. Remember, they will numb your throat and dull oral pleasure and taste. A full stomach also heightens the gag reflex. I'm not telling you to starve yourself before some hot date, but I know one man who covered his partner in a banquet of shrimp lo mein because he just had to take that extra inch!

Now some advice for the penetrator. If your partner is skittish or prone to gagging, let him control the oral sex. It's his mouth and his gag reflex. When you ram your penis in or force him to take it all, you're sure to make him gag or, worse yet, bite down. Force during oral sex propels your penis to the back of his throat and stimulates gagging. Your penis covers his windpipe and he feels like he is suffocating. Panic sets in—and that's not conducive to good sex. Most men enjoy fellatio as long as they don't feel threatened.

If the very idea of going down on you is not something your partner relishes, then talk about it but don't force him. Find out what it is he doesn't like. If he criticizes your hygiene, then instead of getting embarrassed and defensive, listen to what he has to say and discuss what you can do about it. Your groin is covered with bacteria and sweat glands. While some men find natural odors a turn-on, they are not everyone's cup of tea. If you have a fungal infection (jock itch or crotch rot), get rid of it before questioning your partner's devotion. A hot shower or bath taken together and a strategically placed dab of cologne can also heighten desire.

And be responsive to your partner's needs. Contrary to

what you may believe, he wasn't placed on this earth just to suck your penis. (Well, maybe he was.) After a while his jaw muscles fatigue, and if you force him to keep going, it hurts. Although you may want to believe that the mere presence of your penis in his mouth is stimulation enough to keep him aroused, it may not be. Don't forget his sexual needs, and use your hands or your own mouth to keep him turned on too. The same holds true even if you're the one on your knees; your mouth may not be stimulating enough. Sure it is at the beginning, but after a while your partner may get bored. Use your tongue and lips to heighten his pleasure. Pay particular attention to stimulating the sensitive frenulum at the base of his glans. (See Figure 8.2.) Be careful your teeth or scratchy beard don't irritate or cut his sensitive skin. Your five o'clock shadow may look hot in a bar, but in bed it can burn.

And use your hands. So his penis is in your mouth; it doesn't mean that your hands are on vacation. Let them roam over his body hunting out his most sensitive spots. Your hand can be an effective mouth extension, keeping you from gagging while at the same time driving him wild.

But is fellatio safe? That is the question that every gay man loses sleep over. Maybe your partner came in your mouth or maybe he had so much pre-cum that now you're worried that you're at risk. I wish I could give you a straightforward answer that yes, oral sex is 100 percent safe or no, it's not, but I can't. Researchers have proven definitively that unprotected anal sex and intravenous drug use are the two highest-risk behaviors that transmit HIV. We also know that the risk for HIV infection rises in proportion to the number of different sexual partners you've had. So if we know all this, why don't we know if oral sex is safe? When HIV first exploded, scientists frantically searched to find causes. Surveys explored gay sexual practices at a time of unsurpassed sexual freedom. Virtually everyone who tested positive for HIV related a history of numerous un-protected oral and anal sexual encounters. This made sepa-rating risks impossible.

Research in the late 1980s focused on detailing sexual practices of HIV-negative men who later became positive. Doctors hoped that by doing so, they would learn if men who practiced oral but not anal sex contracted HIV. Sounds fine, but the numbers of HIV-negative gay men who had only oral sex and still became positive was fairly low, mak-ing statistical analysis of risk factors difficult.

Medical literature certainly cites anecdotal cases where HIV infection was presumed to be transmitted through oral sex, but isolated incidents do not provide an answer with any kind of certainty. Most scientific studies that looked at HIV transmission through oral sex failed to document a significant rate of HIV infection. Although some men be-lieve they contracted HIV from oral sex, transmission rates are essentially no different from those of men who also deny unprotected anal sex. I know it sounds illogical, but men questioned about sexual practices lie. As one research study showed, many men surveyed by medical personnel were too embarrassed to admit to having unprotected anal sex; thus it appears that these men were infected after seem-ingly safe sex when in fact unprotected anal sex was the more likely route.

A large medical study looking at men in San Francisco concluded that there is a risk of HIV infection after oral sex but that it is much lower than with receptive anal sex. Surprisingly, this study also found that ejaculation into your mouth did not increase risk. This does not mean that it's safe to allow anyone to come in your mouth. As with many things in medicine, you can find data supporting both sides of the HIV/oral sex argument.

Suffice it to say that most physicians agree that there is a slight risk of HIV infection after unprotected oral sex and that the risk increases if your partner ejaculates into your mouth or if you have sores or bleeding gums. One of my patients explained that he doesn't brush his teeth for an entire day before a night of cruising. Obviously his hope is that by avoiding brushing, he will also avoid creating sores on sensitive gums. Although this sounds like a good idea (he does use mouthwash), in practice, most oral sores implicated in HIV infection are very tiny, *chronic* irritations at the gum line and they are present whether you brush or not. We don't know if not brushing affords you any additional protection.

Condoms clearly reduce the already low but possible risk of HIV transmission during fellatio, and the Centers for Disease Control recommends using condoms for all oral sex. Clearly, most HIV enters your mouth as part of your partner's semen, but don't forget that his pre-cum contains virus as well. Unprotected oral sex even without ejaculation may not be safe enough. If your HIV-positive partner is rough and injures your throat, he can increase your chances of infection. Some men believe that not swallowing a partner's semen decreases their chances of HIV infection. Probably not true—especially if they let semen sit in their mouth exposed to oral sores while they run to the bathroom. Acid in the stomach kills HIV and makes infection almost impossible. So swallowing or not swallowing has very little effect on HIV transmission—the main risk occurs when he ejaculates into your mouth. One final warning: Although the risk of contracting HIV via oral sex is low, it undoubtedly increases in direct proportion to the number of different penises you suck and the number of men who ejaculate into your mouth.

HIV isn't the only STD you can catch during oral sex. Just about any STD present in one partner can be transmitted to the other during unprotected oral sex with or without ejaculation. (See Chapters 3 and 4.) An oral STD is harder to diagnose, because the symptoms may be very different from those of a genital infection or can mimic other non-STD conditions (such as an ordinary sore throat). Doctors are also less likely to think of an oral STD infection unless you tell them that you've had unprotected oral sex. A condom is protective, but often it isn't used during fellatio without ejaculation. In addition to preventing STDs, condoms during oral sex may help a nervous partner enjoy sucking your penis more. Not only will he feel more protected, he might also enjoy the taste if you use a flavored brand.

The oral-insertive partner is also at increased risk for developing urinary tract infections, urethritis, prostatitis, and epididymitis. (See Chapter 8.) Your partner's mouth is a veritable garden of bacteria that, through prolonged or repeated oral sex, can travel down your urethra, causing infections.

I have treated men with nasty penile cuts and scrapes from teeth. You might enjoy a little bite during oral sex that, as passions rise, becomes too strong. If your partner draws blood, however, immediately stop and wash your wound thoroughly with an antibacterial soap. Hydrogen peroxide is also a good cleanser because it helps kill oral bacteria. Any antibiotic cream, such as Bacitracin or Neosporin, works well and should be applied at least three times a day after thorough cleansing. If your wound reddens, swells, or begins to hurt, consult your doctor immediately.

We've all heard the emergency room stories about men brought in with one hand clutching their groin while the other holds a jar containing what's left of their penis. Can this happen? Of course it can. I've seen it once in a man who pushed in so deep that his partner began choking. When he wouldn't pull out he left his partner no choice. (It was meant as a warning bite.) When a man thinks he is choking, all rational thought disappears. If biting down is his only way to get a penis out of his mouth, then bite he will. I have also heard of a patient whose partner bit his penis off because he had a seizure during oral sex. If you do find yourself in this horrible predicament, go immediately to an emergency room with your severed anatomy wrapped in a wet cloth on ice. Doctors can try to surgically reattach your penis.

Before moving on, it is important to address water sports. Allowing your partner to urinate on you is safe provided you don't have any open cuts or sores. Although urine most often is sterile, urinary tract infections, prostatitis, epididymitis, and other genital STDs, including HIV, also infect urine. Any of these infections can be transmitted unwittingly should your partner's infected urine come in contact with your blood through an open sore.

Other unwanted complications can arise from drinking urine. Urination rids the body of excess substances and dangerous wastes. When you drink a man's urine, your body digests it, absorbing it into your own bloodstream. (No, it just doesn't pass right out of you.) While many of these substances and wastes, such as sodium, potassium, nitrogen, and ammonia, are not dangerous to healthy people, they can cause serious complications to those with kidney, liver, or heart disease. As an example: Men with high blood pressure must limit their salt intake. If your lover's urine is full of sodium, drinking it can raise your blood pressure dangerously. A word of advice: Before you drink up, consult your physician to make sure you're healthy.

Anilingus

Whether it's called anilingus, rimming, or anal/oral sex, the very thought of it turns off some people, while it's a totally hot sexual act for others. The skin around your anus extending out to your scrotum and buttocks is rich with sensory nerve endings that, when stimulated by a finger or tongue, come alive with pleasure. These nerves also cause reflex twitching of anal sphincters and further heighten pleasure. Anilingus can be a prelude to anal intercourse or just an extension of fellatio as your mouth drifts posterior.

As with any sexual act, a clean partner is definitely a plus. Some men like to douche or use a gentle enema before anilingus, but as with anal sex, liquid that isn't completely evacuated can seep out, causing even more of a mess. I recommend wiping your anal area with a moist, soft cloth or medicated pad such as Tucks. Wet toilet paper flakes apart and leaves unwanted bits around your anus, which your partner's tongue will definitely not find pleasing. Whatever you use, don't wipe too hard. This isn't the kitchen floor, and you're not Cinderella! Your anal skin is extremely sensitive, and any irritation will spoil sexual pleasure. Tiny cuts or abrasions also can become infected, so be gentle, because no matter how hard you scrub it's still going to be just an asshole and not a banquet table. Don't forget that you can also take charge and wash your partner if he isn't as clean as you'd like. Just don't embarrass him in the process. If you're in the shower as a prelude to sex, don't push irritating soap into his anal canal.

Avoid perfumes around your anus unless you know you're not allergic. Most contain alcohol, which stings, and they can cause anal itching. If you use a massage oil as part of foreplay, rubbing it between your partner's cheeks will certainly make his anus smell better, but the taste may be surprisingly bad and oils can irritate him. As with penises, some men like to rub something sweet (honey or jam) around their opening to create a pleasant smell and taste. Avoid oil-based food products or aromatic oils that weaken condoms in case you proceed to anal intercourse.

If you've resisted anilingus but sense it is important to your partner, you have two options: You can always refuse (that is your right), or you can take a deep breath and dive in. You'll find it easier if you avoid his anal opening at first, concentrating instead on his buttocks and the space between his scrotum and anus. If you get into it, and you probably will, his anal opening will become nothing more than a natural progression of your lovemaking

Your partner may be too embarrassed to tell you that he wants you to rim him. Always be mindful of nonverbal cues during sex. If you find him arching his back, raising his legs in the air, or gently nudging your head lower while you're sucking away on his penis, take the hint. He's probably not going to ask. If it's your first time, tell him, so that he can help you through it. If you're the one trying to get your partner to dive in, be understanding. Force only turns him away. Make sure you're clean, and try a little honey or jam to sweeten the experience.

Fingers can injure sensitive tissues in his anal area. Your tongue, however, won't do any damage. It is soft and pliable and won't tear sphincters or anal skin. But beware of tongue, lip, and chin piercings or a scratchy beard, which can cause nasty scrapes and cuts.

So now that we've discussed the finer points of munching on your boyfriend's tushy, is it safe? As far as the risk of HIV transmission is concerned, anilingus represents a *very* low-risk activity. Clearly if you bite a partner who is HIV positive *and* take his blood into your mouth *and* you have an open sore in your mouth, you can catch the virus. Of course, there are a lot of "ands" in this equation, making your risk quite low. I have not seen a case of documented anilingus HIV transmission in the medical literature, but there are men who catch the virus and deny anal sex. How did they get it? Probably they're lying about abstaining from anal sex or maybe they did get it from anilingus. For now it is best to think of anilingus as probably safe but still with a slight chance of transmitting HIV.

Anilingus can pass virtually any other STD, though, and as we saw in earlier chapters, these STDs, while not carrying the same grave prognosis as AIDS, can be debilitating. And if you get one in your mouth (gonorrhea, herpes, or condyloma, to name just a few), the likelihood that your doctor will make the correct diagnosis is small. So before you go for the old "tongue in cheek," as my friend likes to call it, take a good look and make sure your partner is free of any cuts or discharge.

Hepatitis A and B can both be transmitted by anilingus, and your partner may be contagious before he even knows he's sick. It is questionable whether hepatitis C can be transmitted in this manner.

Like hepatitis, parasites and bacteria are frequent infectious complications of anilingus, and your partner may not exhibit any outward symptoms. Most often these infections produce diarrhea, which can be profuse and debilitating. Giardia and amebiasis are the most common parasitic illnesses transmitted through rimming, while salmonella, shigella, and campylobacter are the most common intestinal bacterial pathogens.

Amebiasis or amebic dysentery, as it is frequently called, is caused by the parasite *Entamoeba histolytica*. It is found most commonly in Third World countries where clean water and proper sanitation are frequent problems. In the United States, amebiasis is seen among immigrant populations who carry the disease from their homeland. Gay men are also frequent targets of parasites because they pass between partners during anilingus. The parasite resides in your colon and either it or its reproductive cysts wash out in your stool. If your partner ingests the organism, it will grow in his colon. Unfortunately, most men infected with parasites are not symptomatic and unwittingly pass them to their partners. Symptoms, when they occur, include crampy abdominal pain, diarrhea (frequently bloody), and

a low-grade fever. In its most severe state, diarrhea and colitis can be severe, leading to death if untreated. On rare
occasions, the parasite can break out of the colon and travel
to the liver, where abscesses develop.

Amebiasis is diagnosed when either a blood test is positive for parasite antibodies or a purged fecal sample (after
laxatives) demonstrates the parasite. The antibiotic metronidazole (Flagyl) cures the infection.

Giardiasis is another parasitic infection passed between
partners during anilingus. Caused by the parasite *Giardia
lamblia,* it is the most common parasitic infection in the
United States. Unlike amebiasis, giardia resides in the small
intestine, and not the colon. Parasitic cysts leave the body
in your stool and can be ingested by your partner. Although
many men are symptom free, common complaints include
upper abdominal pain, nausea, and nonbloody diarrhea. A
doctor diagnoses this parasite by sending you to a laboratory
for an examination of your stool after you have taken laxatives. As with amebiasis, metronidazole cures the infection.

Although infectious bacterial diarrhea from salmonella,
shigella, and campylobacter occur most frequently after in-
gesting contaminated foods (undercooked eggs, poultry,
meats, and dairy products), they also can be passed between
partners during anilingus. Bacteria invade your colon, multiply, and cause diarrhea (sometimes bloody), crampy pain,
fever, and vomiting. Although these infections are usually
self-limited (go away even without treatment), in severe
cases and in men with AIDS, antibiotics are often necessary.
A doctor makes the diagnosis by stool culture, but frequently the diarrhea resolves or you've already been treated
by the time the culture comes back positive. Ciprofloxacin
(Cipro) is a good antibiotic when treatment is necessary.
The downside to routine antibiotic therapy is that while
you feel better quicker, it can lead to a prolonged carrier

state. Carriers are people who feel fine yet shed live bacteria in their stool and have the potential of infecting others.

Some "safe-sex" experts advise using some form of barrier for anilingus. Whether it's a piece of plastic wrap, a cut-open condom, or a dental dam, place the barrier over your partner's hole and enjoy. Unfortunately, the barrier significantly reduces your enjoyment and his. People who like anilingus like its taste, smell, and feel, all of which are sorely altered by a piece of latex or plastic. In the end, men often discard the shield long before oral sex is complete, so they lose any protection. If you want to rim your partner, understand the risks and do your best to ensure he's clean. For most men, using a barrier is probably not a feasible solution.

Before closing our discussion of oral sex, we must talk about our mouths. In addition to possibly harboring STDs that can be passed during kissing (yes, it's a form of oral sex), fellatio, and anilingus, our mouths are full of potentially dangerous bacteria, which become a real problem if you are into biting. Gentle nipping is fine, *but don't break your partner's skin!* If you feel your partner's nipping intensify as passions rise, pull his head away and tell him it hurts. Often he isn't even aware of how much pressure his teeth apply. If he persists, you may want to stop the proceedings. A human bite is more dangerous than a dog's. (Your mouth has more bacteria.) The wound must be thoroughly cleansed (use hydrogen peroxide), and antibiotics (ointments or tablets) are often necessary. If pain, redness, or swelling develops, see your doctor.

Kissing is theoretically a potential avenue for HIV transmission. No case has ever been reported in the medical literature, but doctors continue to issue warnings that deep kissing (whatever that means) still carries some risk. If your mouth is full of sores or if your HIV-positive partner bites you, then you may be in danger of catching HIV. In one early AIDS pamphlet I remember seeing an advisory to use a barrier even when kissing. Forget about it—the only thing you're likely to do is suffocate your partner or yourself.

Summary

Oral sex is enjoyable but encompasses a wide range of activities. Whether it is safe or not depends on where along the spectrum your proclivities lie.

- Fellatio is fairly low risk—especially if you use a condom and avoid ejaculation.
- The Centers for Disease Control recommends condom use for oral sex, with or without ejaculation.
- HIV is not the only STD that can be transmitted during oral sex.
- An STD in your mouth is often difficult for doctors to diagnose.
- Urine may not be sterile. HIV is present in urine.
- Anilingus probably poses little risk for HIV transmission.
- Hepatitis, infectious diarrhea, parasites, and other STDs can be passed between partners during anilingus.
- No case of HIV transmission from kissing has ever been documented.
- A human bite is dangerous and needs medical attention.

CHAPTER 10

Monogamy or
Promiscuity?—

OR DO WE HAVE TO CHOOSE?

Every *medical evaluation begins with a thorough history.*

"Do you have protected sex?" I asked the young man seated before me.

"I never let anyone fuck me unless I really know them."

"But is it always protected?"

"The kind of guys I sleep with are clean. I'm negative. And what does all this have to do with a hemorrhoid? That's what's killing me."

My questions made him edgy, but they had to be asked. "What about other STDs?"

"What else is there besides HIV? Like I told you, the guys I sleep with are clean. I don't go to bathhouses."

He still didn't believe me the following week when I called to tell him his anal culture for herpes was positive.

Men are not by nature monogamous creatures. Biologically males of most species spread their semen to whoever will take it. Monogamy is primarily an intellectual and emotional state. For some gay men it represents the ultimate in any relationship between two loving partners, while for others the mere notion of any sort of couplehood sounds too much like a heterosexual marriage. "That's not what being gay means," they argue, believing that safe-sex teaching and a push toward monogamy as a means to thwart the AIDS epidemic has dealt a serious blow to "gay" culture.

For me, my sexual practice does not define me as a gay man. It is definitely a part of my "gayness," but it is not the sum total of my being. I believe that choosing a monogamous relationship does not make you less gay. Humans are social creatures, and many of us search for a mate with whom we can share our lives. This does not mean that you are trying to emulate a heterosexual existence, it just means that you want a partner. The key is to know what is best for *you*. Don't be swayed by what others think.

And gay men deal with issues that our heterosexual counterparts never face. We would never tell an HIV-negative straight couple to continue having safe sex (except for purposes of birth control) once they enter a monogamous relationship. And yet gay men are advised to do this all the time. Why? Because HIV is far more prevalent among men who have sex with men, and men are promiscuous creatures. Monogamy takes a concerted effort. No decision to abandon safe sex between gay partners can be made lightly. The cost of a mistake can be lethal.

Medical research has documented that gay men in relationships are more likely to have unprotected anal sex than men who are not in relationships, whether they are monogamous or not. Obviously, this is a potentially very dangerous situation. We also know that almost half of all gay men in relationships who engage in unprotected sex do not know either their or their partner's HIV status. Again, this is high-risk behavior. Gay men in relationships may be lulled into a false sense of security that has no basis in reality. They wrongly assume that by virtue of their couplehood they are protected from HIV. Knowledge about partners'

HIV status, sexual behavior, and commitment is our only defense.

For many gay men the issue of monogamy is a moot point because they are unattached and actively dating. Sure, the idea of a long-term relationship sounds appealing, but so far they haven't found the guy. Dating by its very nature is not monogamous, and few of us date one man at a time. Each date you go on brings with it questions regarding whether you will have sex with the guy and if you do how far you'll go. And lurking in the back of your mind is that old fear: Will this be the one who gives you an STD? There are ways for us to protect ourselves from HIV and STDs as long as we're willing to make the effort.

Whom You Sleep With

Whether you're monogamous or not, the only way absolutely to prevent catching an STD is to not have sex at all—including kissing. Even that guy you're seeing could give you something like herpes months into your relationship because he had a flare-up. For most of us, giving up sex is an unacceptable notion. We see someone hot, someone we're attracted to, and desire kicks in, sometimes clouding judgment to the point where it can't be trusted. (Especially if we're under the influence of some drug or alcohol.) (See Chapter 11.) In previous chapters I have tried to lay the framework for you to make a sound decision about whom you have sex with. If you know the risks and what to look for, I can't guarantee that you will never catch an STD—they are just too prevalent in this day and age— but at least you'll be armed with the knowledge to make the best possible choice. Many of us carry the hope of one day living that storybook life with our own Prince Charming. But we forget that we have to kiss a lot of frogs before we find our prince. Kissing frogs is not a problem as long as we know our own limitations and those of the frogs!

When AIDS first happened upon the gay world, numerous studies analyzed the sexual practices of gays. Staggering numbers of sexual encounters coupled with orgiastic group sex seemed the rule, not the exception. Even under the shadow of AIDS, many of us still have sexual histories numbering in the hundreds or even thousands, but we remain free of HIV. Clearly, safe sex has made the biggest difference, but so too has our growing understanding of various STDs. The guidelines issued by the Centers for Disease Control on how to avoid contracting HIV include the warning against having sex with an infected partner. For many gay men, this is unacceptable. It is fine to have sex, to experiment and to love—just do it safely and with the strength of knowledge.

Where you find "love" has a lot to do with how great your risk is for catching an STD. The more sexual encounters your partner has had, the more likely he is to bring an STD into your relationship. Now, I certainly don't expect you to demand a list of his previous conquests, but there are clues. If your dream boy is lying naked on a bed in some bathhouse begging you to enter, or hanging out in a steam room flashing his erection, chances are he's not a virgin and you're not his first. Although it should go without saying that prostitutes expose themselves to numerous partners and as such are the most likely to give you more than an orgasm, I am amazed by the number of patients I see who are shocked to learn they caught something from a call boy.

As one patient told me, "I'm too busy to waste time on idle chitchat. I work twelve-hour days, then spend another two at the gym. When I'm horny I call someone from the ads. They're always hot, and I know I'll get what I want. They have to be clean. It's their business."

212

Sure, he got what he wanted from his last experience, but he also got herpes as his lasting reminder.

I know you can find true love in a bathhouse, and I'm not telling you that all men there carry STDs, just understand what you're getting into. The kind of sex your partner usually has and the type of sex you have with him helps predict your risk for catching a new STD. Even if the guy is just "servicing" you, don't be shocked if you catch something from his mouth. Faced with an unknown partner in a high-risk situation, mutual masturbation is safe and can be hot.

Try talking to a potential partner before bedding him. Straightforward questions like "Am I your first tonight?" or "What STDs have you had?" certainly work but will probably scare him off. And even if he sticks around to answer your questions, there is no guarantee that he'll tell you the truth. Less direct questions often will provide the same information within the framework of a normal conversation and not make you sound so much like the sex police. Ask what he likes sexually to get a clue as to how high risk his behavior is. (Does he like to get fucked, even without condoms? Does he routinely let men come in his mouth?) A person's drug history also has bearing on his chance of carrying an STD. Men who have sex while under the influence are prone to sexual carelessness. The number of previous partners a man has had also impacts on his risk for carrying an STD. Has he ever been in a relationship? Have his relationships been measured in weeks, months, or years? While not a guarantee, a man who dates or has had lengthy relationships is probably lower risk than someone who *just* frequents bathhouses or other high-risk environments.

If you find taking this sort of sexual history before you remove your clothes embarrassing, remember that your prospective partner is probably just as nervous as you. No one wants to catch an STD, and it is in the back of every dating guy's mind. Ask a question and chances are he won't be offended, and it might just open up a dialogue you both find interesting.

I know some men who, in lieu of asking sexual history–type questions, try to estimate their risk by checking a prospective partner's home for various telltale medications. One patient said that on going home with a new guy, he would immediately ask to use the bathroom. Once safely behind the locked door he ran water to camouflage the noise of the opening medicine cabinet door. If the medicine cabinet was clean he'd ask for a drink of ice water. That necessitated a trip to the kitchen, where countertops, windowsills, and usually the refrigerator could be perused for those little pharmacy bottles.

Sure, you'll probably find out if your prospective partner is HIV positive, provided he's on medication, but you certainly won't know if he just had a shot for gonorrhea or if he hasn't seen a doctor for that nasty discharge. You won't be able to detect most STDs by a quick search for medicine bottles. Many times even an infected partner is unaware of his condition because he is symptom free or has delayed seeing a doctor hoping his problem will just go away.

Besides analyzing your risk of catching something from a new sexual partner, you must know your own limitations as well. Are you the kind of guy who can go to a "jerk-off" club and just jerk off? Or will you be down on your knees in a flash or bent over in a dark corner while some guy whose name you don't even know plows away? Can you call a talk line and just talk? Are you drunk or drugged out of your mind before you find yourself in some guy's bed? Your own behavior probably has as much to do with your relative risk of catching an STD as the guy you sleep with.

So you've asked some questions and you've decided that you want to have sex with the guy—well, not so fast. Any good doctor will tell you that a history is only half of an evaluation; don't forget the physical exam. Surprised by this notion? Why shouldn't you examine any prospective partner before performing the most intimate of acts? When in some exotic new restaurant, you smell your food, look at it closely before tasting that first bite, don't you? So why shouldn't you do the same with a new partner before he winds up in your mouth?

I don't expect you to don a white coat and rubber gloves, but at least give him the once-over *with the lights on!* Don't make it a clinical examination, make it a hot sexual experience, and *keep your eyes open.* (See Figure 10.1.) Be aware of any sores on his penis, and if you see one, ask about it. Don't be embarrassed; you have a right to know what you're exposing yourself to. And don't forget to look in his pubic hair and scrotum, other harbingers of STDs that aren't covered even if he wears a condom. Tiny clustered open sores or blisters can mean herpes, and you might catch it just from jerking off. A larger open wound certainly can be from an overzealous previous conquest, but it may be from syphilis, not teeth. When a partner has penile sores, it's best to limit contact (hands without cuts are usually okay) until you know for sure. Be careful that you don't touch your penis when touching his. Small bumps especially on the undersurface of his penis can be hair follicles. Warts tend to be flatter and have broader bases, while follicles look like the goose bumps you get when you're cold. Hair follicles are usually the same color as surrounding skin, whereas warts may be either lighter or darker.

If your date seems to have an inordinate amount of precum or if his testicles are tender when you gently rub them, think about the possibility of urethritis, prostatitis, or epidi-

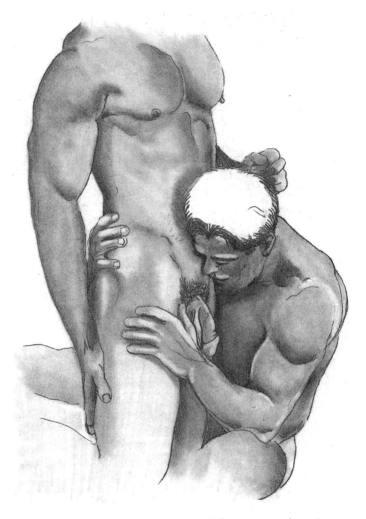

Figure 10.1: Examine your partner before sex. It can be erotic.

dymitis. These are also contagious, but you'll probably be okay if you limit the session to masturbation. Again, don't forget to wash your hands before touching your own body.

I've talked about masturbation quite a bit as being relatively low risk. It is, especially if the masturbation involves two naked guys touching only their own dicks. Even if you do him and he does you, and you both wash your hands after it's all over, you're probably pretty safe and it can be very hot. The minute it goes beyond that with your penis rubbing against his, docking, or rubbing between butt cheeks, your risk rises significantly. And once body cavities are entered, risks climb further. Now, I'm not telling you "Don't suck his cock" or "Don't let him suck yours." Just use your brain. If he's got a lot of pre-cum and you're worried, or if he's got some sore that *might* be from his zipper, put a condom over it and you'll probably be fine.

An anus—whether his or yours—is the area most at risk for STDs. If you don't know the guy, it may be best to stay away. In any case, the same applies to his anus as it did to his penis—keep the lights on, your eyes open, and look first.

Don't expect the skin around his anus to be as smooth as what you see on guys in porn magazines or movies. Skin tags or external hemorrhoids are present in about half of all Americans and are easily confused with warts. While hemorrhoids generally arise from the anal opening and extend outward as a continuous piece of flesh, warts are often scattered around the opening. If it's fleshy and more than half an inch from the opening and doesn't look like a pimple, consider it a wart until proven otherwise. If you are worried about catching something from his anus, stay away. If you can't stay away, or even if you are sure that he's clean, always *wear a condom.* Even if you're just rubbing on the outside and penetration is the farthest thing from your mind, *wear a condom.* I can't say it enough: Rubbing with-

217

out penetration or ejaculation is often enough to transmit most STDs. Although a condom is your best protection, it still doesn't cover a man's pubic hair, the base of his shaft, or his scrotum, all potential sites for men to carry or catch many STDs.

I've spent time telling you what to look for in him, but don't forget to let him examine you. You're probably thinking that you know you're clean, but don't be so sure. While it certainly is difficult for us to examine our own anuses, it is something a partner can do easily. If he asks you about something, *don't be offended.* Answer him and remember he has just as much right to protect himself from STDs as you do. He may even be freer to allow your inspection of him if he knows you expect him to do the same to you. Remember, you're probably *both* afraid of catching something. The fact that he's also cautious makes him a less risky sexual partner.

So how do you make it a sexual experience and not a medical examination? Romantic music certainly helps, massage and other aromatic oils are nice, and so is a lot of kissing while you look. A shower scene is totally hot, and while you're washing his most intimate spots, check him out.

I'm sure you're aware of how your doctor's touch is different from a lover's, but you don't have to touch like a doctor to get similar information. Gently work your hands over his penis and through his pubic hair while looking for little nasties. Even if you see something worrisome, you probably won't catch what he's got from this brief contact if you follow it by thorough hand washing. You can always work on his thighs or lower abdomen (low-risk places that are often quite sensual) with your hands and mouth while conducting your STD inspection. Not only will you whip him into the desired frenzy, but chances are you'll be swept along as well. Don't rush. Take your time pleasuring him in low-risk kinds of ways while completing your survey. Your doctor's exam may take only minutes, but neither of you anticipates an orgasm by the end.

Gay men fear HIV transmission most often during sex, and rightfully so. But sometimes we don't fear it enough. Medical research documents the high frequency of men having unprotected sexual encounters—including anal sex with ejaculation. What I've tried to do in this text is alert you to the myriad of other STDs as well. I've told you which warning signs to look for in a partner with regard to many other diseases but not HIV. The reason for this is simple. It is often impossible to tell that a prospective partner carries the virus. Sure, we've all seen men in end stages of AIDS, but thankfully that scenario is growing less common as medicine makes great strides in HIV treatment. Temporal wasting (sunken canyons on the sides of his head) and dark-purple blotches from Kaposi's sarcoma are now often the exception instead of the rule. In short, there is no way to tell if a prospective partner has HIV unless he tells you. Given that fact, the best alternative is to be safe. Fortunately, HIV is still fairly difficult to transmit without exchanging semen during anal or possibly oral sex or via shared needles. Using a condom and a little intelligence is often protection enough.

You've checked him out, he's clean, and you embark on a hot sexual experience. Make sure you use condoms. In a recent survey conducted in Philadelphia, almost half of the men who'd had unprotected anal sex did so because the sex was too exciting to bother with condoms. Almost another third gave their partner's refusal to wear one as a reason for unprotected anal sex. Poor excuses. Unroll the condom on him—that can be hot too. If he refuses, tell him your life isn't worth the risk.

After you have sex, what should you do? Take off your condom and throw it away. Make sure he does the same.

Immediately after you've come during anal sex, withdraw holding your condom tight. Any loss of erection loosens the seal and semen can spill out. And after he's ejaculated, don't let him rub his penis against your anus. He'll still discharge semen for a while, and if the head of his penis is against your anus, it can seep inside. This is especially true as more time passes after ejaculation, because prostate enzymes work to liquefy his semen, making it much more runny than when it first shot out.

I know it is far more romantic to lie entwined with your partner in a postorgasmic embrace, but if you don't know what he's got, it is probably smarter to excuse yourself and wash off with an antibacterial soap. You have no reason to be embarrassed about trying to protect yourself from an STD, and many can be prevented just by a thorough and immediate washing. You'll do your partner a great service if you drag him along to the bathroom as well. Wash your hands, penis, scrotum, and anus well and don't forget any other area where his cum landed. Towel off and then climb back into bed for postcoital cuddling. You'll sleep a lot more soundly if you know you're clean instead of worrying while his semen drips down your thigh.

You say this guy you're climbing into bed with is a regular fuck buddy and you've got nothing to worry about with him. Wrong! Whether you get together for hot sex once a month or once a week or even once a day (then it's a relationship), you still don't know whom he's slept with in between. Unless you're in a monogamous relationship, there is no excuse for not staying vigilant. You never know when he's going to bring more to your bed than his erection.

What do you do if several days after the most fantastic sexual experience (or even one of your worst) you find yourself staring at a sore on your penis or a ton of pre-cum even when you're not aroused? See your doctor! Don't think it's nothing or try to rationalize it away. Chances are you caught something treatable, and the quicker you see your doctor, the quicker you'll be cured. And just as important, early treatment prevents you from transmitting the STD to someone else. Embarrassment and delay only aggravate your situation and complicate treatment.

Monogamy

He lay down on the exam table, his newly tanned physique a sharp contrast to the white paper. "How was your vacation?" I asked somewhat enviously.

His body tensed. "Fine, really fine," but his expression spoke otherwise.

I tucked my stethoscope back in my pocket and asked if it was something he wanted to talk about.

"We went to a club," he began slowly. "Not just a club, a bathhouse."

"Did you both want to go?"

"It seemed like a hot idea. The guys we saw on the beach all day were incredible. We were so whipped. We just went into this big room—a huge jerk-off scene. A lot of groping, nothing more."

"So what's the problem?" I asked.

His eyes remained transfixed by the blood pressure machine on the opposite wall. "Chris, my partner, enjoyed it more."

"By more, you mean more than you or more than you wanted him to?"

He smiled for a moment and then shrugged. "When I looked up and saw this blond guy with Chris going nuts in his hand . . . I didn't like it at all."

Monogamy is not for everyone, and sexual experiences outside of a relationship are not inherently wrong—provided both partners agree. What is wrong is cheating.

The word "cheating" implies deception, and that is exactly what occurs when you have sex outside of your relationship without telling your partner. Whether you call it polyamory, an open relationship, or a ménage à trois, the key must be honesty. Your partner has a right to know that you are having sex with others. In this day and age, the risks of sex outside of a relationship are more than emotional—a partner who cheats can bring home a deadly disease. In addition to transmitting HIV, sex in the 1990s has the potential to pass numerous STDs between partners.

Honest communication between partners is key to healthy sexual experiences. No one assumes that sleeping with a man commits you to a monogamous relationship, and until boundaries are set it is best to maintain safe-sex vigilance. When a date becomes more than just a date and you feel the stirrings of a relationship unfold, it is time to begin your sexual dialogue. But remember that a sexual dialogue does not automatically imply a monogamous relationship. You are still free to date and have sex with others if that is what you both choose, but discuss what limitations, if any, are to be set. As I mentioned earlier, not only can certain sexual practices be higher risk than others, so too can partners. Your relationship may be moving toward anal sex (if you haven't already done it) or unprotected sex, and you need to know how risky your partner's sexual practices are with others. Is he having sex with call boys or in other high-risk settings? If he is and this is unacceptable to you, then you can either agree to a new boundary or continue with less risky sex. Some couples draw the line at anal intercourse outside of their relationship but allow masturbation and oral sex, while some view any form of sexual experience with others as forbidden. This is a decision for partners to make together.

When partners agree to be monogamous, they each must have a thorough and identical understanding of what that means. Sex therapists agree that an active fantasy life is healthy for any relationship. If your partner fuels his fantasies with sessions on the Internet, is that a problem for you? Many men in monogamous relationships still masturbate. Most of us have no problem with a partner who looks at a porn video or magazine while stroking away, but how do we feel about phone sex or chat rooms? Does communicating with a stranger you can't touch constitute cheating? And can you trust yourself not to find out where "Mr. Hot" lives and jump in the car for a little rendezvous? These are all questions that men who have sex with men need to address. And just because you think it's fine doesn't mean your partner will agree.

The start of a new relationship is a time for honesty. It never gets easier. We all bring baggage to each new encounter, and I doubt any of us will be virgins by the time we meet Mr. Right. If you worry that having this type of talk might scare your new love away, do your best to reassure him. It is far more dangerous not to have the talk and to assume that he is as faithful as you are. As time passes and your relationship intensifies, it might be even more embarrassing to bring the subject up. You're setting yourself up for heartache if after months of dating you finally summon the courage to discuss sex only to find out that while you assumed you both were faithful, in reality he was screwing around with many other guys.

When broaching the subject of "who else are you sleeping with and what are you doing with them?" it is important not to take a judgmental stand. If your new love senses he'll hurt you with his honesty, he may not tell you what you *need* to hear. Approach the subject with openness, knowing that it is only a jumping-off point. Everything is negotiable. And just as you expect your partner to be honest with you, you must be honest with him. You'll feel far worse admitting that you just gave him gonorrhea if he had

223

no idea you still had fuck buddies on the side. If you don't have this discussion, then your healthiest solution is to maintain safe-sex practices.

Talking in a frank manner at the start of a relationship also opens the door to nonsexual discussions as well. It allows you both to sense how serious and committed you are to each other. While one of you may be dreaming of monogrammed towels, the other might be thinking of his next good time. Any sexual discussion often brings forth these important issues.

Before relaxing your safe-sex policies, determine what STDs your new partner has had or still has—and not just HIV! Herpes will not go away and condyloma probably won't either. Hepatitis B, if chronic, can be passed between partners as HIV can. It is possible to keep from catching an STD from your partner, and knowing if one of you is a carrier helps. Then and only then can you make an educated decision as to whether to continue and what precautions, if any, you're both going to take. If he bolts because of something you admitted, then look on the bright side: It's better that he left early on than after you'd solidified your bonds.

Even though you set sexual boundaries early in your relationship, you probably will want to reevaluate the subject periodically. As relationships strengthen or even deteriorate, what once worked may no longer be applicable. Most couples reach a point in their togetherness when they recognize their commitment to each other—which may or may not imply sexual monogamy. Disagreements must be dealt with. Again, knowledge and honesty are key. If your partner wants you to have sex with only him and you know you can't, then tell him. You may try to give up other men, but be honest if you fail. Therapy can be extremely beneficial as you try to work through differences.

Clearly a truly monogamous relationship is the best protection you have against an STD. Many couples abandon safe sex once they are committed and *both* HIV negative or positive. If you find yourself in a once-monogamous relationship that is no longer working and you've begun to have sex with others, then you must tell your partner. Your fear of admitting the truth puts him at risk as long as he continues to have unprotected sex with you. I know you're thinking that you always wear a condom for anal sex with others, but I hope you've learned by now that there is plenty more you can bring home besides HIV. You might be totally safe and participate only in low-risk activities like mutual masturbation, but low risk does not mean no risk.

Just because your doctor tells you that you have an STD when you know you've been faithful doesn't necessarily mean that your partner strayed. I know it's hard, but try to keep an open mind. Certain STDs can be in *your* body for years and you just never knew you had them. You may have had mild herpes attacks in the past that only now became painful. Urethritis, prostatitis, and many other infections can also be chronic and so mild that you were unaware until you had this recent flare-up. Warts are probably the most common example of STDs that can stay dormant until something triggers an outbreak. Even if your current partner is the only guy who's ever penetrated you, it doesn't mean he's the one who gave you the disease. Fingers, toys, and skin-to-skin contact with prior partners can pass STDs. And the same holds true for your partner. If he did give you the STD, he might have had it for years but been unaware. His flare-up could make him suddenly more contagious and able to pass it on to you. So before you point a finger (or anything else), remember, a new STD doesn't prove cheating, and *you* might have been the one to bring it to your relationship.

For some couples, sexual monogamy is not the answer. They have sex with other partners, or a couple might have sex with others in a three- or foursome (or even more). One patient I treat routinely goes to a bathhouse with his lover of many years and they take separate rooms, have separate experiences, and then leave together at an appointed hour. Most couples in open relationships know that each is free to have sex outside of their relationship, but this doesn't lessen their commitment. Again, knowledge and honesty will keep you physically and mentally healthy. You must set boundaries that you both adhere to. If you agree to have other partners, then discuss what is allowed. You might draw the line at anal sex or forbid frequenting high-risk places. You know the risk of each type of sexual behavior, and you must decide how far you'll both go. If your partner does not want you fucking someone else but jerking off is fine, then tell him if you can't respect his wishes. If he's on his back with his legs in the air, he has a right to know that you haven't had high-risk anal sex with others.

I have a patient who tells me that anytime a relationship goes beyond the third date he insists that they both get HIV-tested. Even if his new boyfriend tells him he's negative, my patient wants to know for sure. Moreover, he wants to be able to reassure his boyfriend that he is negative as well. This isn't to imply that my patient wouldn't date anyone who is positive; he has. He wants to know so that he can come to the relationship knowing how stringent his safe-sex practices will be. If a lover is positive and you are negative, you might not have anal sex or might have oral sex without ejaculation or only if he wears a condom. The point is that you can make your choices only on the basis of knowledge. If you are an HIV-positive man, you have a responsibility to protect your negative partner even if he doesn't wish to be protected.

Although my patient's third-date rule may seem a little

harsh, I agree that it is wise for partners to be tested early on in a relationship. This isn't because I believe that one of you might be lying (although it has happened) but because many men do not realize they have HIV. Many couples relax their safe-sex practices as their relationship progresses, something that you may not want to happen if one or both of you is positive. As mentioned, men who are HIV positive have a higher likelihood of carrying other STDs and may even have resistant strains of HIV that can pass between partners.

I also advise couples in long-term relationships to undergo periodic HIV testing to be sure that neither one has become infected. It is best to have a set date each year (an anniversary or birthday is easy) so that suspicions of infidelity are not raised should one partner come home and suggest that they both be tested.

I treated a man who first came to me with herpes, which he picked up while having *protected* anal sex in a bathhouse. A few months later he returned to my office with molluscum—also from a bathhouse. When he came in with condyloma (guess where he got it?), he finally admitted that his relationship with his lover wasn't working. (Hello?) Anal sex was very important for my patient, and his partner refused to fulfill this sexual need. Rather than discussing it or terminating their relationship he chose to cheat on his partner, having anal sex in bathhouses. I suggested couples therapy, because my patient was allowing a relationship that wasn't working to impact negatively on his health.

No one formula will work for everyone; each relationship is different. Dialogue between partners is crucial, as is honesty. If your situation changes or your needs are not being met, then talk to your lover. If an unhappy partner confronts you, getting defensive will only worsen the situation and terminate any chance at meaningful discussion.

Summary

Sex between men is too dangerous in this day and age to be taken lightly. Keep your sex hot, safe, and honest. Once sexual boundaries are established, they must be respected.

- Monogamy isn't right for everyone.
- Try to assess your relative risk for catching an STD from a potential partner by asking pertinent questions.
- Before having sex, look for signs of STDs. Keep the lights on, your eyes open, and the experience hot.
- If you're worried that he has "something," masturbation is usually safe.
- Wear a condom.
- After sex, wash up with an antibacterial soap.
- You can't usually tell if someone has HIV just by looking at him.
- Discuss sexual boundaries with your partner and work toward an agreement.
- An open relationship is fine as long as you're honest with each other.
- Even men in monogamous relationships should have periodic HIV tests.
- Knowledge and a condom are your best protection against an STD.
- A new STD doesn't have to mean cheating.

CHAPTER 11

Drugs—

OR SHOULDN'T YOU SEE YOUR

PHARMACIST?

I had never seen him before. I glanced down at the intake form all new patients fill out and saw that his complaint was a rash. No, he'd never had it before, and no, he hadn't changed his diet or switched laundry detergents. Every question I asked searching for possible causes was met with a no.

He lifted his shirt to reveal red blotches covering his torso. "It definitely looks allergic," I said. No telltale scabs to suggest bug bites, and the fact that his genital area was spared made an STD unlikely.

"As I said, Doc, I only eat pure foods, nothing processed. Organic vegetables and fruits, free-range poultry, no meats. I even use hypoallergenic soaps."

"Where'd you get your tan?" I asked before giving up and sending him to a dermatologist.

"The Pines. I have a share there."

I smiled. Now it made sense. "Only organic, natural foods, right?" I asked.

He sighed and gave me a weary nod.

"Well, how about drugs? Use any of them?" His face reddened and I didn't wait for an answer. "Ecstacy, K, poppers?"

He nodded yes to each, and his eyes widened. "You think that's what gave me the rash?"

"I know that's what gave you the rash. You're so fastidious about your diet only to swallow pills filled with garbage every Friday and Saturday night."

"But I gotta dance."

Drug use and abuse has always been prevalent within the gay community. Drugs don't have to be illegal to be abused or addicting. Alcohol and nicotine are legal, while others, including tranquilizers, diet pills, and narcotic pain medications, are controlled and obtained with a doctor's prescription. And all have a high abuse potential. Before discussing each drug individually, let's examine certain principles that apply to each. Although the makeup of "legal" drugs is tightly regulated by the Food and Drug Administration, illegal drugs are not. Most are manufactured in home laboratories and cut with anything from talcum powder to baby laxatives; occasionally the additives are more harmful than the drugs themselves. Inconsistencies with respect to purity and quantity of drug in each tablet or vial also contributes to the danger and unpredictability of illegal drug use. One pill barely touches you, while the next lands you in a coma.

Drugs you take, whether legal or illegal, alter mood and perception by changing chemical balances within your brain. These changes, while producing desired and often pleasurable effects initially, leave your brain depleted of necessary substances when the drug wears off. What started out as a pleasurable ride turns into a nightmare before it's over.

Drugs, whether prescribed or not, can also become addictive, leaving you crippled by something that started out to be just a kick or mood raiser. Addiction often has a biological or genetic basis and begins so gradually that most men don't even know it's happening until it's too late.

Drugs are also a major enemy in our fight to eliminate HIV. By altering chemicals in our brains, drugs distort judgment. What might have been a safe sexual encounter dissolves into reckless abandon as you focus on your high and getting off instead of getting protection. A recent medical survey polled gay men in Philadelphia and asked them why they had unprotected anal sex. Almost a third of men attributed their failure to use condoms to drugs or alcohol. In addition to impairing judgment, drugs can decrease sensation. A sexual act that you might have stopped because of pain is suddenly tolerable. But when the drugs wear off you're left with a bleeding rectum or torn nipple.

Swallowing one pill affects any other pill you've already taken. We call this phenomenon of a medication increasing or diminishing the effectiveness of another a drug interaction. Pharmacists and drug companies keep data banks of potentially dangerous drug interactions and warn you if your doctor prescribes medications that shouldn't be taken together. Fine and good for prescription drugs, but no data bank tells you if the Ecstacy you've just swallowed is going to negate the protease inhibitor you took an hour before. Illegal drugs are not cataloged by dangerous interactions, making combinations a crapshoot. When drugs potentiate each other, a much lower dose can become an overdose.

As we wash down that pill with vodka or beer, most of us forget that alcohol is a potent depressant. If you're already bombed, alcohol in your blood can combine with another drug you take to put you into a life-threatening situation. Something you tolerated in the past may have an entirely different effect after you've been drinking.

In the case of pills, size does not matter. In other words, that tiny pill or small sip can knock you on your ass. Most of us look at a pill and figure it's small, so how much harm can it do? You might even be tempted to try two, only to wind up in some emergency room. Don't be misled because a liquid is clear or a pill is tiny.

A drug's potency depends on how much reaches your

brain and is affected by how you take it. When you inject a drug, the entire amount hits your brain immediately, making even a small dose highly potent. A pill, on the other hand, must be digested, so absorption into your bloodstream is a more gradual process. The amount reaching your brain at any given time is less than when a drug is injected, but its effects last longer. Smoking or snorting also gets a drug into your bloodstream faster than if it's swallowed. Shooting, snorting, or smoking a drug makes it more potent, and as such, your danger of overdosing increases.

Drug use adversely affects your nutritional status and immune system. You skip medications and forget to eat because you're too out of it. You dance right through one dose of your antiviral medication, then sleep through the next. Drug impurities stress your immune system and harm healthy T-cells. Added together, these side effects conspire to make HIV-positive patients susceptible to falling T-cell counts and rising viral loads.

There is a chemical basis to many psychological disorders, and drugs can worsen these conditions. If you're prone to depression and swallow that little pill, you might be nearly suicidal by the time it wears off. Medications prescribed for psychiatric disorders also can have potent interactions with abused drugs. Be careful, because the antidepressant you've recently started may combine with that hit of K and cause an overdose.

Although your typical fantasy image of a gay man may be one who is young, handsome, virile, and impervious to harm, most of us don't fall into that category—and not just because of HIV. We have diabetes, high blood pressure, heart murmurs, and many other medical conditions that you'd never guess from outward appearances. Abused drugs affect many other organs besides our brain. In addition to your glorious high, that pill might raise your blood pressure to dangerous levels, stress your heart with rapid or irregular beats, or poison your kidneys. If you already have medical problems, the added stress can be enough to tip you over the edge.

Alcohol

Yes, alcohol is a drug—the most widely abused drug in this country! Although it may feel otherwise, alcohol is actually a depressant and anesthetic. When you take a drink, your stomach and intestines rapidly absorb the alcohol. As it reaches your brain, alcohol slows nerve impulses, at first eliminating your inhibitions. As blood levels rise, you may feel happy and garrulous, but you lose the ability to perform complex neurological functions. Your balance falters and you have difficulty walking, dizziness, slurred speech. You might even find yourself in a sexual situation you would otherwise have avoided. Continued drinking slows your breathing, and you can slip from stuporous sleep into a coma. Your danger increases when the depressant effects of alcohol combine with the same properties in other medications. Alcohol and narcotics are a particularly deadly combination, because together they can stop your breathing.

As we all know, you're likely to experience what is commonly referred to as a hangover the morning after a night of heavy drinking. You feel tired and depressed, and your head won't stop pounding. Dehydration is common because your body needs water to break down the alcohol.

Alcohol is metabolized by your liver, and heavy abuse can cause dangerous inflammation called alcoholic hepatitis. With long-term abuse some men develop cirrhosis and liver failure. Alcohol can adversely affect other medications broken down by your liver (such as protease inhibitors) and damage many other organs, including your stomach (causing ulcers or gastritis) and pancreas (pancreatitis).

Alcohol's abuse potential is great, and unfortunately there are no clear-cut boundaries among social, moderate, or problem drinking. Alcoholism develops insidiously, with the victim often the last to know. The task of steering him to treatment usually falls on friends and loved ones. There are no easy ways to tell a partner that he is a substance abuser, and he probably won't listen. Prepare to bear the brunt of his anger as he struggles to come to terms with his addiction. You'll *both* need help. Fortunately, excellent programs like AA (Alcoholics Anonymous) and Al-Anon (for partners of alcoholics) have made great strides in controlling the impulse to drink.

Cocaine

Manufactured from cocoa leaves, cocaine can be snorted, injected, and even smoked (crack). When mixed with heroin and injected intravenously, it is called speed-balling. In its medical form (that's right, doctors prescribe it), cocaine is a potent anesthetic and it constricts blood vessels. Many ear-nose-and-throat specialists use it to shrink and anesthetize swollen nasal passages before operating in that area. Once cocaine enters the bloodstream, it blocks nerves in your brain from taking up the potent chemicals dopamine, norepinephrine, and serotonin. Doctors have identified two distinct phases of a cocaine "high." Phase 1 is characterized by an initial rush of euphoria accompanied by insomnia, anorexia, and in some men hallucinations and paranoia. When your hallucinations become tactile you have what is commonly called the cocaine bugs. In addition to affecting your neurological system, cocaine also raises your blood pressure and pulse, occasionally to dangerous levels. In phase 2 cocaine can cause irregular heartbeats, heart attacks, seizures, and stroke.

After a coke binge you enter a withdrawal state, which is essentially the opposite of your high—euphoria is replaced by a depression that can lead to suicidal thoughts. You might also experience periods of binge eating and sleeping. Your withdrawal lasts far longer than your high, sometimes stretching for several days. In addition to suffering dangerous cardiac effects, long-term cocaine abusers often destroy their nasal passages and may have lingering psychological disturbances. Cocaine is definitely addicting.

Amphetamines

Amphetamines, commonly called speed, are similar in chemical structure to dopamine (a brain chemical essential to nerve transmission). Like cocaine, amphetamines, whether injected, smoked, or snorted, produce an initial state of euphoria, insomnia, and hyperactivity replaced by depression (even to the point of suicide) and marked need for sleep during withdrawal. Crystal, a commonly abused amphetamine, also causes rapid heartbeats and may lead to addiction. Men who use crystal say that it makes them horny, but beware: Impotence or a poor erection are just as common.

MDMA, a synthetic amphetamine better known as Ecstacy, is extremely prevalent in the gay community. For many men it is the fuel that keeps them dancing all night long, as they feel happy and less inhibited. They find themselves able to talk to strangers they otherwise would have thought unapproachable. Unfortunately, Ecstacy is often viewed as harmless when in fact it can be quite dangerous. In addition to producing desired euphoria, tremors, insomnia, and sweating are frequent side effects. While dancing the night away in a hot club you could sweat yourself into serious dehydration. Take too much Ecstacy and you expose yourself to dangerous irregular heartbeats, seizures, stroke, or hyperthermia (too high body temperature). As with any drug, when you land from your glorious high, no doubt you'll find yourself at the opposite end of the emotional spectrum; the dancing queen who'd talk to anyone is a bitched-out, depressed, exhausted monster the morning after—and it can take two days to recover while your brain slowly replaces depleted chemicals. Medical research has shown that prolonged use can lead to permanent destruction of brain cells, and Ecstacy also can have dangerous interactions with other medications. Beware of combining Ecstacy with Prozac or MAO (monoamine oxidase) inhibitors, another class of antidepressants. There are even reports of death after taking Ecstacy with a protease inhibitor.

Sedative Hypnotics

This class of drugs includes barbiturates and the all-popular benzodiazepines, with Valium and Xanax the poster children. Although many hypnotics are not illegal and often are obtained by prescription, their abuse potential is great. Men approach multiple doctors for prescriptions and sell them to friends. An internist may give you a script not knowing that your psychiatrist has as well.

Hypnotics work by affecting the GABA system of the brain, which controls three functions: sedation, anxiety, and the prevention of seizures. Thus the drug you take dissolves your troubles, leaving you calm and free of inhibition. In high doses, hypnotics put you to sleep, slur your speech, or occasionally make you violent (especially in combination with other drugs). Although most commonly taken in tablet form, liquid preparations for injection are also prevalent. The half-life of these drugs (length of time they hang around in your body) varies greatly. Valium has one of the longest half-lives, while Xanax has one of the shortest. These medications are highly addictive. Withdrawal from them can produce nausea, tremors, irritability, seizures, hallucinations, rapid pulse, and high blood pressure. Flumazenil (Romazicon) is an antidote for overdose.

K, or Special K, as it is sometimes called, is another potent hypnotic that is actually a disassociative anesthetic used frequently in surgery. So how does that fit in with your night on the dance floor? K, or ketamine, as it is known in the medical community, makes your brain feel disconnected from the rest of your body. Some men find this quite pleasurable—as if they are floating above their body looking down—but for others it is a disturbing kind of high bordering on feeling psychotic. Take too much and you're catatonic and ready for surgery—or at least the hospital. Although sold in a liquid form that can be injected, most often K is boiled down to a powder residue and then snorted or swallowed. Sexually, K can make it seem like the guy fucking you without the condom is fucking someone else, and you're just there to watch. I warn you: If HIV is passed, it will be *you* who gets it, not the guy floating above you. Doctors worry about the potential for serious yet still unidentified side effects from prolonged K abuse (including personality changes).

GHB is another abused hypnotic, but potentially it is far more dangerous than the others because there is very little difference between the amount you need to feel high and the amount that puts you into a coma. In other words, there is little margin for error between enough and too much—especially if you're mixing it with other depressants, like alcohol or Valium. Because GHB is a clear liquid, most men mix it with water and swig it on the dance floor. For some reason, people perceive anything clear as harmless, and you never know how much drug you're getting when you drink up. Combine all this with the fact that you can easily overdose on GHB and you're courting an extremely dangerous situation.

Vasodilators

Poppers, or amyl nitrite, are the most commonly abused of the vasodilators. They produce their high by expanding blood vessels so that your heart races as your blood pressure drops—you swoon, get dizzy, the room spins—like "almost" fainting. Although your rush lasts only moments, it comes as your heart struggles to keep blood flowing to your brain. Amyl nitrite is sold as a liquid, but you inhale the fumes to get high. These fumes are quite flammable, so beware of smoking and doing poppers at the same time. The liquid itself can burn the skin around your nose. In men with heart trouble or blocked arteries, poppers can lower blood pressure to the point where the brain and heart can't get enough oxygen. Recently deaths occurred in men who combined poppers with Viagra. Both drugs dilate blood vessels, and, together, they can drop blood pressure to lethal levels. Headaches are another bad side effect of poppers—especially with repeated use, as men try to maintain the fleeting high they get from each sniff.

Narcotics

Synthesized from poppies, opium became man's first narcotic, used widely not only for its unparalleled euphoria but also because it eliminated pain. Morphine, heroin, Dilaudid, and Codeine are natural drugs made from poppies; most others, including Demerol, Darvon, Percocet, and Percodan, are synthetic. The list of synthetic narcotics is endless, and varies by strength as well as the substance they are combined with. (Percocet contains Tylenol, while Percodan contains aspirin.) Heroin, like all narcotics, is highly addicting. Some gay men believe that if you snort a narcotic it is not as addicting—wrong!!! These drugs are just as addicting whether swallowed, injected, smoked, or snorted. Once addicted to heroin, people find it is so nearly impossible to break free that therapy often centers on control (methadone) rather than kicking the habit.

In addition to producing euphoria, narcotics deaden pain, diminish libido, and depress your respiratory and heart function. In high doses, narcotics will stop your breathing (an overdose). Narcotics are vital in providing pain relief after injury, surgery, and many other debilitating conditions, such as cancer. If you suffer from a chronic pain problem, keep in mind the addictive potential of narcotics and the fact that tolerance builds with prolonged use. Consider using alternative medications, such as nonsteroidal anti-inflammatory drugs (NSAIDs), which are highly effective and not habit forming. If you require narcotic pain medication but your supply outlasts your need, throw away any extra pills. Keeping drugs around only entices you or others to abuse them for that little pick-me-up. It's easy to convince yourself that your muscle ache requires Percocet when Tylenol would do just fine. If a loved one has severe pain from incurable cancer, don't be afraid to give narcotics, because pain control is essential and the addictive potential doesn't really matter.

If you've had a problem with drug abuse in the past (even if it's alcohol), you probably have what is termed an addictive personality. If at some future point you require pain medication, help yourself by admitting your problem to your doctor. Ask for a NSAID-type medication. If it isn't strong enough you may require narcotics, and there is nothing wrong with that. Don't be embarrassed by your past problem, and ask your doctor for a narcotic to get you through a period of terrible pain. Medications serve a valuable purpose when used properly. To safeguard against addiction, request a limited supply and throw away any extra the moment you can switch to something milder.

Hallucinogens

The name may sound dangerous, a class of drugs you would never try, until you remember that marijuana is actually a hallucinogen. LSD and mescaline are certainly far more potent, but all of these drugs are capable of producing hallucinations. Marijuana in low doses causes a high similar to what you'd expect after a few drinks of alcohol, but if you smoke a lot, hallucinations similar to those from LSD are possible. Although your auditory acuity is said to increase with marijuana and other hallucinogens, true auditory hallucinations are rare. Most men describe visual alterations in both form and color. If marijuana is smoked, the high begins within minutes and lasts for two to three hours. When you eat marijuana, onset is more gradual, but because 50 percent of the active drug is destroyed by smoking, you get a much greater high from eating the same amount of grass. Tolerance to hallucinogens builds rapidly with repeated abuse. Blood or urine tests detect evidence of marijuana use for as long as two weeks. Remember this if your job mandates drug screening. Medically, marijuana stimulates your appetite, is a strong anti-emetic (keeps you from vomiting), and is effective in treating certain forms of glaucoma. Although activists are campaigning to change laws, marijuana is still illegal in this country.

Psychosocial Aspects of Drug Dependency

I glanced at my patient's intake sheet and saw nothing to explain his visit. I treated his lover for years, but never him. "From the looks of everything you seem fine," I said. "Is this a routine checkup?"

He shook his head. "I'm fine. It's about Bill."

I shifted in my seat. I never like to discuss one patient with another—even if they're lovers. "Then maybe we need to discuss this with Bill too."

"He doesn't believe he's got a drug problem. He said I'm exaggerating. Trust me, I'm not exaggerating. He'll listen to you. I know he will."

"Look, I'm here for you both, but don't be so sure he'll listen to me." I looked at my calendar. "Can you get him to come in tomorrow?"

"No, we're flying to Miami. It's the White Party."

Not everyone who drinks or uses drugs has a problem. In fact, most don't. There clearly is a biological and possibly even genetic basis to addiction. And for those in relationships, drug dependency is not an individual problem; it is a couples problem with the nondependent partner playing an integral role. Any solution to a partner's drug problem becomes a couples solution, with both men taking active roles.

No one wants to believe he has a drug problem. We all try to explain and rationalize it away—anything to keep from facing the truth. Partners do the same thing. They never want to believe their lover is addicted. If you've got a drug problem, expect to hear about it from friends long before you recognize it in yourself. If someone tells you he suspects you have a problem, listen. He's probably right.

If friends remark that your personality has changed, it's probably from drugs. It can begin as episodic outbursts when you had always been even-tempered. Little problems you could have laughed off in the past suddenly take on paramount importance. Every struggle becomes a do-or-die battle. You fight with everyone and break old friendships. Watch for other erratic behaviors, including interrupted sleep and spending sprees.

Depression is another very common symptom of a drug problem. It is especially common after a period of prolonged drug use while your brain struggles to replenish vital chemicals. You may not get out of bed—except to go party some more. You miss work and other critical appointments—but always have a good excuse. And it was never your fault; someone else is always to blame.

You may also notice physical symptoms of your growing drug troubles. Weight loss or weight gain are common, as are frequent headaches. Check your arms and legs. Are they covered with unexplained bruises? You probably got them when you fell down, stoned out of your mind. Watch your blood pressure, because it can fluctuate with drug use.

Now take a hard look at when you use drugs. Try to keep track of patterns. Are you using drugs every day, spending more and more money to get high? Once you take that first hit, do you have trouble saying no? If the answers are yes, get help. When you go over your list of times you got high, try to remember the reason. People with drug dependency always find excuses to explain why they got high. Maybe your day was too hard and you needed to unwind. Maybe you were owed. Or your day was great and you wanted to celebrate. No, you *deserved* to celebrate. Some men need drugs to relax, while others need them to sleep. When you hear your reasons and they all sound too familiar, get help.

Last, look at your own family. If a parent or other close relative had a problem, you may have one too. Most people with drug dependency can easily point to a relative with the same trouble. Our parents taught us well, and if they taught us about alcohol and other drug dependencies, it may be impossible to avoid those same pitfalls—especially when our genes pull us in that direction.

If your partner has a drug problem, you must share the burden. Many psychologists use the term "enabler" to describe a person who helps his partner, often subconsciously, maintain a pattern of destructive drug use. You may handle drugs and alcohol fine and enjoy getting high. You do a little coke after work and your partner does a little coke. He willingly accompanies you to every circuit party and does every drug you do. But he's got a problem, and your drug use perpetuates his.

You're probably always "cleaning up" after your partner's binges, explaining why he missed work or that important appointment. Sure, you're helping him out of a difficult spot, but he needs to feel the consequences of his actions if you expect him to change. Drugs feel great. No one gives them up unless they realize the harm they're doing.

Enablers may encourage a partner's drug use for more personal reasons. If your partner is stoned, you may find it easier to control him. When high, some men drift into their own world, and you get a welcome break from a difficult lover. Some men use drugs for sexual seduction. If he can get it up only with a little Ecstacy, you're probably only too happy to pass it his way.

Often enablers use their partner's drug problem to keep themselves out of the spotlight. If drugs turn your lover into the life of the party, you're freed from holding up your end of the conversation. If most of your relationship revolves around discussions of *his* drug problems, then it deflects attention from what is really wrong with the relationship and your own shortcomings. Your drug-dependent partner becomes an easy target. Everyone wants to talk about him and everyone offers you, the suffering spouse, support. It's a comfortable situation for someone afraid to examine his own issues.

Getting your lover help may be impossible, and many psychologists recommend that *you* get help first. Learn how drugs affect your partner and your relationship and what you're doing to perpetuate his use. Any good therapist will help you steer your partner toward treatment, and it won't be easy. You'll bear the brunt of his anger, and it may be hard to take all the shit he dishes out. Al-Anon offers excellent support groups for partners of addicted people. You can't do it alone, so give them a call.

Former First Lady Betty Ford brought drug dependency into the rarefied world of the rich and beautiful. No longer a problem of lower socioeconomic groups, it almost became fashionable to admit to a stay at her clinic. (Just imagine how quick you'd perk up party conversation dropping the little tidbit that Liza was in your group.) Fortunately, gay men now have their own clinics specializing in drug and alcohol dependency and mental health. Pride Institute, based in Minnesota with satellites in New York, New Jersey, Illinois, and Florida, and Alternatives in California are just two examples. Check with your doctor or gay-specific classifieds to find other organizations, locations, and contact phone numbers. Make the call. It's hard, but it's the first step in your new direction.

Summary

Drugs and alcohol have always been prevalent in the gay community. They are major obstacles in our efforts to eliminate HIV. Abuse potential is high, and drugs don't have to be illegal to be dangerous.

- There are no standards for illegal drugs, and composition varies widely.
- Drugs alter chemicals in your brain, so what starts off as a pleasurable ride often dissolves into a nightmare before it's over.
- Addiction or dependency begins gradually, and most men don't realize they have a problem until it's too late.
- Drugs distort judgment, making safe sex less likely.
- Drugs (alcohol included) can have harmful interactions.

- Snorting, shooting, or smoking a drug makes a smaller dose more potent.
- Drugs affect many other organs besides the brain.
- If a partner is a substance abuser, you both need help.
- If you have an addictive personality, let your doctor know.
- Narcotics are sometimes necessary even if you've had drug problems in the past.
- Marijuana is still illegal in the United States.

CHAPTER **12**

How Do I Find a Doctor?—

OR YES, THEY'RE EVEN IN PEORIA

I had been struggling with my own sexuality for quite some time, and I had not yet come out on a professional level. In the midst of my emotional turmoil I developed a Bell's palsy, or paralysis of one side of my face. Being a physician, I immediately thought the worst and assumed I was in the midst of a lethal stroke. I sought emergency medical attention from a well-respected colleague of mine. The doctor, although not gay, had a reputation of being gay-friendly. Like many gay men who hide their sexuality, I struggled with whether I should admit my homosexuality to the doctor. I knew that in rare instances Bell's palsy could result from AIDS and my sexuality might be important. In the end I vowed to finally tell the truth.

"Come on in, Steve," he called out across a room crowded with patients. His warmth was genuine. He tapped my cheek and pronounced "Bell's palsy" even before we reached the examining room.

"Are you sure that's all it is?" I asked as I edged up onto the table.

"Pretty sure, but let's do this right. First a medical history, then a complete exam. We're going to pretend you're a patient and not a doctor."

This was fine with me. When doctors get sick, all of their medi-

cal training goes right out the window. I wanted him to pretend I knew nothing—which at the moment was absolutely true.

He asked straightforward questions regarding my drooping cheek and unblinking eye before moving on to an inventory of illnesses I'd had in the past. So far my sexuality remained hidden, and I kept looking for an opening to bring it up in case he never asked. When he closed my chart and tucked his pen into his breast pocket, I thought he'd finished asking questions. I cleared my throat and took a deep breath of courage. I was going to admit something for the first time.

The tone in his voice as he said "And of course you're not gay" stopped me cold.

I laughed with him while once again listening to the latest "fag" joke—for the last time. He took care of me that day and then I found a new doctor, someone who was gay-friendly not only in practice but in heart.

Medical care is changing, and so are doctors' perceptions of homosexuality. Although the AIDS epidemic has done great harm to the gay community, it has also accomplished some good. In addition to mobilizing us into a cohesive political force that can no longer be ignored, it ushered in an era of gay medicine. For the first time physicians were paying attention to gays as a unique group with our own unique problems and needs, in ways previously reserved for the elderly (geriatric medicine), women (women's health), and adolescents as a subset of pediatrics. True, gay health-care initially focused on AIDS, but out of that grew AIDS prevention and healthcare directed at wellness instead of illness.

AIDS forced gay men out of the closet and forced doctors to realize that many of the "normal" men they had treated for years were, in fact, gay—and it made no difference at all. We learned that if it was okay to walk into a doctor's office as an openly gay man to be treated for AIDS, it was also okay to walk into that same office to be treated for the flu or high blood pressure or any other problem. The difference was that now we could be treated under an umbrella of honesty—both with ourselves and our physicians.

Not only has the AIDS epidemic liberated gay patients from this medical closet, it has also liberated healthcare workers. Suddenly AIDS allowed physicians to admit their own homosexuality, with many finding their vocation treating gay men and women—and not just for AIDS. We see openly gay plastic surgeons (who needs more work than a queen?), dermatologists, surgeons, psychiatrists—specialists in every field of medicine now cater to gay patient populations.

AIDS has also forced insurance companies, health maintenance organizations (HMOs), and numerous other ancillary services to take note of gays. Now domestic partners can obtain health coverage under some plans, and insurance companies in urban centers market to gay communities.

Gay healthcare has made great strides during the AIDS epidemic, and there is no longer any reason to go to a physician with whom you can't be honest about your sexuality.

Gay or Straight, Male or Female

Today many gay men can choose whether to see a male or female doctor and even one who is gay or straight. I am not saying that every gay man should be cared for by a like-minded physician. A straight doctor is certainly capable of treating gay patients in a nonhomophobic environment— just as women have received excellent care from male physicians. The key to any successful doctor-patient relationship is mutual respect and trust. If you have this with your doctor, then it does not matter if it's a he or she, gay or straight.

While your sexuality does not define every medical condition you might someday face, there are certain gay-specific issues that you may need to discuss with your doctor. For instance, your high blood pressure can be treated by any internist, but rectal bleeding after anal sex may be difficult to discuss with a straight doctor—just as it may be difficult for some straight doctors to hear. As we all know, not everyone who seems open and free from homophobia really is. One way to determine if a potential doctor is right for you is to ask friends who have seen him (or her). If they tell you that they never discussed sexual issues, or that when they did, the physician seemed uptight, it is probably best to look elsewhere for care.

By the same token, not every gay physician will be right for you. Gay doctors can be just as homophobic as straight doctors, and the mere fact that they're gay does not mean they dispense quality care. Your doctor's clinical judgment, intelligence, and ability to relate to you are far more important than his or her sex and sexuality.

You also can find a gay or gay-friendly physician through a gay and lesbian switchboard. Many doctors actively court the gay community by listing themselves with these services. Gay-friendly doctors also advertise in local gay-specific magazines or yellow pages. Other than word of mouth (which is probably the best recommendation) these are the most common ways for doctors to reach out to the gay community.

Calling your local hospital to ask for a recommendation is also a good way to find a gay doctor. While the hospital may not specifically maintain a listing of homosexual physicians (although it may), chances are it can tell you who specializes in HIV treatment. The doctor recommended may not be gay, but there is a high probability that whoever it is won't be homophobic. Even if you don't have HIV you probably will be welcomed as a patient.

National hot lines, the Internet, and the Gay and Lesbian Medical Association are other good sources for finding gay or gay-friendly physicians.

If your community has no gay or gay-friendly physicians, find the closest one to consult with on gay-related health issues. It might be worth your while to travel manageable distances on those occasions when you want to discuss a problem you can't tell your local doctor. Even most rural areas have been affected by the HIV epidemic, and you should be able to find someone close by who is at least gay-friendly. I have received phone calls from men around the country with questions they can't ask their community physician. This is one of the few situations when I am not opposed to telephone medicine. Most doctors will answer your questions, tell you if your problem could be related to your sexuality, and try to refer you to someone who can help. So if you can't travel to a doctor you'd feel comfortable with, try picking up the phone and calling. Just don't abandon your community physician, whom you'll want to see for routine medical problems.

What to Look For

There are certain qualities to look for in any physician you choose. And remember that the important phrase is "you choose," because healthcare today is like any other service-oriented industry—it is competitive, and you, the consumer, have the right to make a choice. Even HMOs with strict provider lists usually afford some choice by offering more than one physician in each specialty.

Do not go to a doctor you don't like or can't be honest with. He or she may have the reputation as being the best and the brightest, but it's better to find someone you can relate to on a personal level. Most ordinary medical problems require the services of a *good* doctor, not some world expert who can't look you in the eye. Any good doctor knows when your problem is beyond his or her abilities and will be honest about it. Chances are that situation will never arise.

A big question facing many patients is whether to seek a doctor through a clinic or a private office. Private offices generally offer more personal care and allow for a close relationship with your doctor—but not always. Some practices have become so large that they are nothing more than healthcare factories. For some of us the word "clinic" conjures up images of dirty booths, with desperately ill, indigent patients who wait hours for treatment. While this is the case in many facilities, more and more clinics resemble posh doctor's offices dispensing quality care, and you should not count them out. Stay away from any clinic or doctor's office where you cannot see *one* primary physician at least most of the time. There will be occasions when your doctor is away and you are treated by a covering staff member, but this occurs even in single physician offices. If you see a different doctor at each treatment, you forfeit a chance to forge a strong doctor-patient relationship. This is important, especially when you are being treated for a chronic illness. Not only will your relationships with your many physicians suffer, but so too might your medical care. Each visit with a different doctor necessitates spending time reviewing your chart. If the doctor is rushed, important points might be missed. Any lingering questions may still not be answered, or you'll have to spend valuable time reviewing all that has come before.

Although clinics may lack the personal touch of a private office, many are multispecialty sites where you can see doctors specializing in almost all areas of medicine. This may be a plus if you see a range of different specialists (an internist for high blood pressure, a gastroenterologist for an ulcer, and a plastic surgeon for everything else!).

251

Some clinics are staffed by residents in training from local hospitals, and this may not be what you want. While residents are always supervised by an attending (certified) physician, your primary care is dispensed by a doctor in training. Most residents are excellent physicians and may be more versed in newer methods than more established doctors. Residents, however, train on average for three years and leave, so you'll be reassigned and have to start building a relationship from scratch.

In addition to offering more personal doctor-patient care, a single-physician office or small group practice may foster a closer relationship with other healthcare workers. This may sound like a trivial matter, but many patients rely on smart nurses and secretaries to answer simple questions over the telephone. If office personnel know you, they can expedite paperwork and simple matters like prescription renewals without demanding that you first speak to the doctor. Staff members often can get to the doctor more quickly than you can, and you'll waste less time waiting for medication or that disability check.

Patients on disability (with Medicare insurance) tend to think that a clinic is their only healthcare option. While this may have been true in the past, today most private physicians accept Medicare. If you have Medicare, call the physician you'd like to see and ask if he or she will take your insurance. Don't assume you're relegated to clinics.

Unfortunately, the same is not true for many men on public assistance or welfare. Most private physicians will not accept this type of health coverage because of low reimbursement rates. Still, it's certainly worth a phone call to inquire.

Even if you are treated in a private doctor's office, there may come a time when some of your care is turned over to a nonphysician, usually a physician assistant (P.A.) or nurse practitioner (N.P.). Although not physicians, these highly trained providers are adept at handling routine medical problems. If you want to discuss your problem with the supervising doctor, just ask. Many patients I know have come to rely on nonphysician practitioners for more personal care. In this age of falling reimbursement levels, many doctors make up for lost income by seeing more and more patients. They spend less time with healthier clients and/or hire nurse practitioners and physician assistants to take up the slack. Don't be shocked if your doctor can't see you for that sore throat, blood pressure check, or flu shot. The nurse practitioner or P.A. is well equipped to handle your problem.

You can tell a lot about a doctor by the way his or her office is run. If your phone call gets picked up on the tenth ring by someone who yells "Doctor's office, please hold!" then treats you to ten minutes of Muzak, chances are that the doctor is too busy to give you the time you deserve. If the secretary sounds gruff and uncaring, most likely the doctor will too. The boss, in this case the physician, sets the tone of any office.

When you enter an office for the first time, look around to be sure it's a place where you feel comfortable. Cleanliness is key in any doctor's office, and that is what you must look for. If the place looks like a garbage dump, then the surroundings might be indicative of the care provided.

Look for clues in the office as to whether the place is gay-friendly. While I wouldn't expect to find a Rainbow flag in the waiting room, you might see other indications. Pamphlets addressing gay health issues or gay-oriented magazines might be prominently displayed.

During a patient's first visit, I always talk to him in my consultation room while he is fully dressed. This is a far less threatening environment in which I get to know a patient and find out what is really bothering him. I also don't discuss treatment with a patient while he is shivering in a

253

gown seated on a cold vinyl exam table. I tell him to get dressed and then join me back in my consultation room, where we can talk behind closed doors.

If your doctor tries to talk to you in front of other patients or even in a room with an open door, insist on privacy. Your medical issues are between you and your physician, not anyone else in the office. If your significant other (or anyone else) has accompanied you on the visit, it is certainly your right to request that he join you or *not* join you when you talk with the doctor before and after your exam. But don't expect to have company during your examination. Most doctors, myself included, frown on having an audience other than office personnel.

And what if after your exam you don't like the doctor or the advice? Just because you see a doctor once doesn't mean you have to go back or that you have to follow the instructions. Even if he or she is registered as your primary physician within your health plan, you can always change to someone else.

Telephone medicine is usually not good medicine. If you call for an appointment and your doctor calls in prescriptions instead of seeing you, think about finding someone else. While some problems can be handled by telephone, many should not be. If your doctor refuses to see you despite your belief that you merit a visit, demand an appointment or go somewhere else.

Do I Need a Specialist?

When confronted with a medical situation, it is always best to see your primary care physician: the person who knows you best and is adept at handling a wide variety of ailments. If that doctor feels you need a specialist, a referral will be provided. Do not run to emergency rooms for nonemergency problems. The care they provide is geared to life-threatening situations, is far less personal, and probably is not as thorough as that which a regular doctor provides for more routine problems.

Most primary care specialists can treat STDs. Patients with STDs also often turn to dermatologists first, because so many of these diseases begin as skin rashes. Urologists are also adept at handling most male-related STDs and other genital problems. But again, your primary doctor can treat most of these problems or refer you to a specialist when necessary.

If you are too embarrassed to see your regular doctor about an STD, most cities have clinics specially set up for these diseases. While these are often fine, I urge you to put away your embarrassment and talk to your own doctor. I guarantee you are not his or her first patient to catch this doing that!

As always, if you don't think that your regular doctor is treating your condition properly or if you fail to improve, it is your right to ask for a referral to a specialist or to go for a second opinion. Most doctors welcome second opinions for patients with difficult problems—either to confirm that their treatment plan is correct or to offer a different perspective on a complicated problem.

What do you do if your primary doctor refuses to refer you to a specialist and your insurance company won't let you go without it? Occasionally there is nothing you can do. If your doctor is offering an alternative treatment plan instead of sending you to a specialist, try what is recommended. Many primary doctors are able to handle more than you imagine. For instance, don't be surprised if your primary physician chooses to treat your rash with medication rather than send you immediately to a dermatologist. If it doesn't work, then your primary doctor will make the referral. Getting angry and screaming will do little to enhance the doctor-patient relationship.

If your doctor flat out refuses you a referral and you still want it, most health plans have patient care representatives you can call to lodge a complaint. You also can request another primary healthcare provider, one more willing to give you what you need. Alternatively, most health plans with restrictive referral lists now offer what is commonly termed out-of-network coverage. This entitles you to see any physician without a referral from your primary doctor. But beware; you'll probably have a deductible to meet (which can run hundreds of dollars) followed by only partial reimbursement for charges. Check with your plan first and know what you're getting into. It is always less costly to get a referral or to see a doctor on your plan than to go outside.

As a surgeon, many of my patients come to me by referral from their internists. Other patients come because of family or friend recommendations. I hate it when patients ask me not to tell their primary doctor I saw them because I'm not the surgeon who was recommended. There is nothing wrong with seeing a specialist different from the one your doctor advised. You are not betraying your doctor, but please keep all doctors informed of who is caring for you. Communication among your various physicians is crucial and can't occur if you hide one from the other. Doctors need to discuss your medical situation so that diagnostic steps are not duplicated and treatments are coordinated. Many conditions and treatments impact one another and could cause dangerous consequences if your doctors are unaware. Let your doctors decide when it is important for them to talk.

I treated a patient who had a slight bleeding problem that, although not serious on a day-to-day basis, could have been life threatening during surgery. My patient did not understand the illness and felt that because it never bothered him, there was no need to disclose it. Although he asked me not to call his internist, I refused. Fortunately for my patient, I learned about his blood disorder from his primary doctor and took the necessary steps to ensure that he didn't bleed excessively during surgery. Most patients do not understand what doctors need to learn from one another.

Some gay men also try to keep their HIV status hidden from various specialists. Even if you are sure that your HIV status has no bearing on your treatment, it is important to tell the doctor, because *you* never know.

Doctor Fees

When you call to make an appointment, don't be afraid to ask questions regarding cost and insurance. Remember: You're the consumer. You wouldn't walk into a store and take something from a shelf to the cashier without even looking at the price. (Then again, maybe you would!) Don't let yourself be surprised when you're presented with a huge bill and the secretary points to the sign stating "Payment is expected at the time services are rendered." You should have known this from the time your appointment was scheduled. If the secretary answers your telephone questions regarding usual fees with "It all depends on what the doctor does for you," he or she might be giving the best answer possible. Many times if you see a doctor for a specific problem he or she may want to perform various tests. Some are done in the office and billed at that time, while others are carried out elsewhere. When faced with this type of predicament, try asking the secretary about standard fees for consultations as well as the price for office tests.

If you are a member of a managed care plan or HMO, be sure to ask if your prospective physician participates. If so, you will be responsible for, at most, a small copayment.

If you contact a specialist on your own and determine that he or she is a member of your group plan, check to find out if you need a referral from your primary care doctor in order for the visit to be covered. Some plans require prior approval or else your treatment won't be reimbursed.

If you are not a member of a managed care or HMO plan, then chances are you will be responsible for some portion of your office visit. Many plans typically cover only 75 to 80 percent of reasonable and customary charges. If your plan covers 100 percent, you might think yourself lucky and then be surprised when you still get a bill for a balance owed. How can this be if your plan covers 100 percent? The answer lurks in those three little words, "reasonable and customary." Your plan determines what "reasonable" fee doctors should charge for any given procedure and reimburses accordingly. Your doctor, however, has no obligation to go along with that fee scale. If your doctor charges $100 for a visit but your insurance company said that $80 was a reasonable rate, you'll be billed for the difference. When you call your doctor, inquire about standard fees and then call your insurance carrier to determine if discrepancies exist.

Men frequently find themselves switched into new insurance plans because their employer changed coverage. If your new plan has a restricted provider list, your original primary doctor may not be a member. Unfortunately, usually this means that you need to choose a new primary care physician. This situation is particularly troublesome for patients with chronic illnesses like AIDS who have long-established relationships with their physicians. If your new plan has out-of-network benefits, ask your old doctor if he or she will accept whatever your insurance pays. Many doctors will agree rather than lose you as a patient. Even if your doctor accepts your insurance with the proviso that you cover your deductible, it may be worth it to spend a little money and maintain a relationship that has worked over years rather than switch to someone new.

No matter what type of insurance policy you have, never go to a hospital or emergency room (unless it's a true life-or-death situation) without first checking to be sure that you don't need prior approval. If you go without the required approval, you may be responsible for the entire fee (and it's never cheap)! Whenever you're admitted to a hospital or scheduled for a test or surgery, either call your insurance company yourself or have someone do it for you. Many policies must authorize medical procedures and hospital stays or else they won't cover your bill.

The biggest problem in healthcare today is the large number of uninsured patients. If you have any health insurance whatsoever, you'll probably be able to find a physician who will accept it as full payment (although it may be at a clinic). Many young men have no idea how costly healthcare can be, nor how at risk they are for illness. When we're young we never think about sickness or hospitalization, and often we don't have money to "waste" on health coverage. Some gay men truly can't afford insurance and don't qualify for disability or public assistance. For anyone in this situation, it is imperative that you research fees before you see the doctor. Most won't react kindly to a patient who after treatment suddenly finds that his credit card is maxed out or there's no money to cover a check.

Men without coverage can ask their doctors about payment plans or seek reduced fees. Sliding scale clinics are also available in most areas, where charges are adjusted according to income levels. While your care may not be as personal as you would like, at least it's affordable.

With respect to insurance, it is important to understand the concept of a preexisting condition. Many plans cover you only for health problems dating from the time your policy goes into effect. Thus if you suddenly develop diabetes, all treatment related to diabetes will be covered. If, however, you were treated for diabetes prior to obtaining your policy, you may not be covered for a varying period of time (usually six to eighteen months, depending on your policy). Not all health plans have preexisting condition clauses (the more expensive ones usually don't, nor do some employee group plans), and documented prior treatment of your problem is usually what insurance companies look for. Thus if you knew you had a hernia for a year before you obtained health insurance, but never saw a doctor for it, you'll probably be okay. Your insurance company will, however, contact any doctors you saw in the past to be sure that there was no prior record of the hernia. Avoid unexpected bills by contacting your insurance carrier to be sure a planned treatment is covered and that there is no preexisting condition clause.

A preexisting condition clause is nullified if you prove that you had continuous insurance coverage before switching to your new plan. This is important to anyone with a chronic illness, such as AIDS. If you've been covered under one plan for several years and then switch health insurance (many times it is because of a job change), your AIDS will not be considered preexisting as long as your prior coverage never lapsed. If you lose your job, you can continue your health coverage through a COBRA plan. This entitles you to pay your premiums directly to the company and maintain your benefits even though you're no longer an employee. You can do this for eighteen months; by then you probably will have found a new job offering health coverage. Your continuous coverage prevents a preexisting condition clause from taking effect. It's expensive to continue a policy on your own, and when you're out of work it may not seem worth it. But if you have a chronic medical problem, in the long run you'll be glad you did. Medicare and public assistance–based health insurances do not have preexisting condition clauses.

When faced with bills from a doctor or other healthcare provider, don't think they'll just go away. Most often medical billing, whether from a doctor or a hospital, is computer generated, and after a certain number of ignored payment requests, you'll be sent to a collection agency. This can destroy your credit rating and set you up for unnecessary legal expenses. Most doctors contract their billing to services and are unaware that you're being harassed for payment. Call your doctor and explain your reason for nonpayment. It never hurts to try, and your doctor might reduce your balance or wipe it out completely. Partial payments through an installment plan, no matter how small, generally will keep collection agencies at bay. If your doctor sent you to another doctor or facility that is hounding you for balance payment, talk to your primary physician about it. He might be inclined to plead your case, and the other doctor might be more willing to listen.

Summary

Healthcare in the 1990s has become increasingly complicated. Insurance rules and regulations change constantly, and the doctor you saw last week may not be in your plan the next. Do your research before going for an appointment so you're not surprised by high fees and large balances. If at all possible, maintain your health coverage even if you have to pay for it out of pocket. You never know when you'll need it. And never put off seeing a doctor because you think you can't afford it. Your health is too important, and there is always someplace you can go.

◈ Healthcare is your right.

◈ Find a physician you can relate to and forge an honest patient-doctor relationship.

◈ If you are unhappy with your physician or the advice, change to someone else.

◈ Always find out your doctor's fees before you visit, and check to be sure your insurance will cover it.

◈ Don't be afraid to ask for a reduction in fees.

◈ Before going to a specialist or emergency room, check to be sure that you don't need a referral from your primary doctor.

◈ Your insurance company may not pay for care related to preexisting conditions.

◈ Medicare and public assistance–based health plans do not have preexisting condition clauses.

The Ten Most Frequently Asked Questions

I always use a condom, so how did I get this?

Always??? Most men would like to believe that they always use a condom when, in fact, on occasion they slip up. Drugs and alcohol impair judgment and are the biggest deterrents to safe sex. When some pill, powder, or liquid whips you into a sexual frenzy, you think only about getting off instead of getting protection. During one of these exceptions to your strict I-always-use-a-condom rule you can catch an STD.

Men who use condoms also pick up STDs in other ways. A condom won't cover your partner's scrotum or pubic region (unless he wraps himself in a garbage bag), and STDs lurking there can spread from his body to yours. Many STDs, including herpes, genital warts, and crabs, require only the kind of close skin-to-skin contact most men enjoy. Sure you use a condom for penetration, but up until that point, rubbing and fondling can deposit little nasties all over your body. Fingers and toys also carry STDs between partners.

Unfortunately, STDs are so prevalent that total abstinence is your only sure way to prevent catching one.

Do I have to see a doctor just because I have rectal bleeding?

Rectal bleeding is a potentially serious problem. Most men notice it after a bowel movement, either on toilet paper or in the bowl. Although rectal bleeding most often results from hemorrhoids, it also can be a sign of other more dangerous conditions, such as cancer or colitis. Try treating slight bleeding that stops soon after your bowel movement with stool softeners (see Chapter 2) and soaks in a warm tub. When bleeding persists for more than a day or two or continues long after your bowel movement is finished, see your doctor. Dark-red or maroon rectal bleeding or associated symptoms such as pain, fever, or pressure in your rectum are far more serious and merit immediate evaluation by your doctor.

Do I have to tell a partner I've had herpes or genital warts?

Herpes and warts are very common and nothing to be embarrassed about. I always advise honesty with partners, especially during a genital wart or herpes outbreak when you are highly contagious. When warts or herpes blisters are limited to your anus, your penis might be safe for masturbation or oral sex. Unfortunately, even if your treated warts or herpes went away, you may still be infectious. Condoms are fairly protective but must be worn from the start of close physical contact. Always wash your hands and any areas where semen lands immediately after sex, and tell your partner to do the same. Soap and water can go a long way toward eliminating many STDs before they take hold.

If I am HIV negative, should I have sex with a positive partner?

Although the Centers for Disease Control advises HIV-negative men *against* all sex with HIV-infected partners, many gay men have it safely. Knowledge is key. Know your risks and make your decision accordingly. Masturbation is safe, but keep his semen away from any cuts or sores on your body. If your HIV-positive partner wants to penetrate you (mouth or anus), make him wear a condom. Many physicians and HIV experts warn against "deep tongue kissing," but there has never been a documented case of HIV transmission from it. If you have HIV, you must protect your partner even if he doesn't want it.

How can I make my penis larger?

You probably can't. When erect, the average penis really is 6 inches long and 1.3 inches in diameter. (Get out those rulers.) When soft, penis size has much greater variability. And as we all know, you can never predict how big it's going to get when it gets hard. Cock rings and pumps help some men add a little length to their penis by drawing in more blood and keeping it there, but priapism (inability to lose your erection) is a danger. (And imagine how thrilled your partner will be while he waits for you to "inflate" your dick!) Penis-enlarging operations are dangerous with often disappointing and possibly disfiguring results. Viagra and other medications designed to treat impotence may make your erection stiffer, but they won't increase size over what you normally have.

What if I get hard while my doctor examines me?

It happens, and there is nothing you can do about it. My advice is to ignore it, and your doctor probably will too. I guarantee that you are not the first person who got hard in his exam room. Some men find their doctor's touch arousing (especially if he's poking around your anus or penis), and some may even be attracted to their physicians. Some apologize for their erections, but it isn't necessary. If you feel you must say something, try making light of it. Humor will help relax you, and Mr. Happy might just go back to sleep. Please don't ask your doctor for a date, because that puts you both in an awkward and potentially unethical situation.

Is it dangerous to put big toys into my rectum, and will it diminish sensation?

Big toys or fisting can be dangerous. Any stiff, long object may not negotiate the natural bend in your colon and tear through the wall—an extremely dangerous situation that requires emergency surgery to repair. Thick toys (especially fists) can damage your sphincter muscle and may eventually lead to an inability to control your bowels. When choosing a toy, make sure it's soft and pliable. And always use common sense: If it hurts, don't force it in.

Anal stimulation has a strong psychological component, and some men find that large toys satisfy them both emotionally and physically. If you find a partner who can't compete with what you have stored in your closet, you may not find him fulfilling. Even if you're used to large toys, most penises will need to stretch you for penetration and this should still feel pleasurable. You might, however, reach the point where you really need to feel opened to the limit for satisfaction, and most men can't do it for you.

Can a doctor tell I've been fucked?

Usually not. A penis stretches your sphincter during anal sex, but it usually regains its tone (strength) soon after your partner pulls out. So unless you're in the habit of going to the doctor right after sex, he or she probably won't find anything other than a normal sphincter. Fisting and large toys, however, can stretch your sphincter sufficiently so that your doctor senses a difference.

I always advise honesty with your physician when answering questions regarding your sexuality and anal sex—especially if you have a problem "back there." Anal intercourse exposes you to many STDs and potential medical problems that your doctor might not think of unless he or she knows you've partaken in those delights.

Is oral sex safe?

That depends entirely on your definition of "safe." When most men talk about "safe," they refer only to their risk of catching HIV. But that isn't enough. Oral sex (even kissing) can pass most STDs, including herpes, syphilis, gonorrhea, genital warts, hepatitis, and urethritis, between partners *without* ejaculation. Sure, you may not catch HIV, but you might take away something other than his phone number from the experience.

Fellatio is relatively low risk for HIV—especially if your partner doesn't ejaculate into your mouth. There have been suspected cases of HIV infection after oral sex, so to be truly safe, insist partners wear condoms. Spitting out semen after a partner comes in your mouth probably doesn't add protection, because your greatest risk occurs when his semen bathes your gums and oral tissues. Some men also believe not brushing their teeth before oral sex protects them from HIV, but I have never seen research to support or refute this conclusion. I believe that not brushing offers no added protection, because tiny sores are always present around your gums from chronic irritation and poor dental hygiene.

Rimming carries almost no risk of HIV transmission, but again you can catch other infections, including diarrhea and hepatitis, from it.

Who's that cute guy in your waiting room?

Don't ask, because your doctor's not going to tell. It's unethical for a doctor to discuss another patient's condition with you—even if you want only his name. If you plan to hit on someone you see in the waiting room, don't expect your doctor to help.

Common Symptoms and Possible Causes

Rectal Bleeding

ANAL FISSURE (TEAR): Bright-red blood streaking stool or on toilet paper and often painful bowel movements.

COLITIS: Bright-red blood or mucus with bowel movements and possible crampy pain. Can be related to bacterial infection or antibiotic use.

COLON TUMORS: Cancerous or noncancerous growths can cause bright-red blood with bowel movements. Pain is usually not present.

HEMORRHOIDS: Bright-red blood on toilet paper or dripping into bowl. Usually painless.

INJURY: Bright-red blood after anal sex or instrumentation. Pain is variable.

Anal Pain

ANAL FISSURE (TEAR): Pain with bowel movements with or without blood, frequently beginning after constipation.

ANAL SPHINCTER SPASM: Severe, sharp pain frequently after a hard bowel movement, forced anal sex, or instrumentation.

FISTULA-IN-ANO: A tubular connection from the inside of your rectum to the outside that causes pain with or without fever. Your pain typically increases in severity until the fistula pops and a small amount of pus or blood discharges.

THROMBOSED HEMORRHOID: Painful, tender, swollen lump adjacent to your anus caused by a blood clot in your hemorrhoid. Bleeding may or may not be present.

TRAUMA: An injury producing pain after anal sex or instrumentation. Bleeding may or may not be present.

Diarrhea

BACTERIAL INFECTION: Associated with crampy abdominal pain after eating spoiled or undercooked food (particularly milk products, eggs, chicken, and ground beef). Also occurs after rimming. Blood mixed with diarrhea may be present.

GASTROENTERITIS: Frequently stomach flu—like symptoms caused by a virus with crampy abdominal pain, fever, nausea, and vomiting.

IRRITABLE BOWEL: "Nervous stomach" with bouts of diarrhea and constipation associated with mood changes and anxiety.

PARASITES: Associated with travel to foreign countries and HIV infection. Crampy abdominal pain and fever may or may not be present.

Penile Discharge

GONOCOCCAL URETHRITIS: Gonorrhea often produces a profuse infected discharge. Burning on urination may or may not be present.

NGU (NONGONOCOCCAL URETHRITIS): Often a clear discharge that can be profuse or visible only if you milk your penis.

PRE-CUM: Begins during sexual excitement when the prostate, seminal vesicles, and smaller accessory glands secrete clear fluid into the urethra.

Testicular Pain

EPIDIDYMITIS: Inflammation of the epididymis behind the testicle. Fever is common.

HERNIA: A hole in the muscle of the abdominal wall. You notice a lump coming from your groin, which may travel into your scrotum. Sometimes you can push it back in. A painful hernia is an emergency.

PROSTATITIS: Inflammation of the prostate that often produces a heavy or painful sensation in the lower rectum. Fever is common.

TESTICULAR TORSION: A twisting of a testicle. Severe pain that begins suddenly and the testicle rides higher in the scrotum. An emergency situation.

VARICOCELE: Enlarged veins around a testicle that cause a heaviness in the scrotum and the squishy feeling of a "nest of worms" above the testicle. Often associated with an increased risk of infertility.

Average Incubation Periods for Common STDs

CONDYLOMA ACUMINATUM (GENITAL WARTS): Average incubation time after close physical contact with an infected partner is thought to be approximately three months but can be as short as six weeks or as long as many years. Many men who have sex with men carry this virus, but they may not have warts. The infection may be incurable.

GONORRHEA: An infected discharge begins two to five days after sex with an infected partner. Pain is common for urethral infections but may be absent in anal infections.

HEPATITIS: Typically you are infectious and can pass the virus to partners before you know you have it yourself. Incubation periods from infection until the time you become ill vary, with hepatitis A averaging two to six weeks and hepatitis B and C averaging two weeks to six months.

HERPES: Approximately one week after close physical contact with an infected partner, a burning sensation begins. A day or two later a small cluster of blisters erupts. Recurrent attacks are common, and the disease is incurable.

HIV: Symptoms of AIDS often don't begin until ten years after infection. Standard HIV antibody tests are often positive two months after infection but can take as long as six months. Viral load measurements sometimes can document infection within one month after exposure.

MOLLUSCUM CONTAGIOSUM: Within one to three months after close physical contact with an infected partner, pin-size pimples with a central depression appear. If untreated, they can continue to enlarge.

NONGONOCOCCAL URETHRITIS (NGU): A clear or infected penile discharge begins one to five weeks after sex with an infected partner. You might experience burning with urination. Untreated infection can spread to your prostate and epididymis.

PEDICULOSIS PUBIS (CRABS): Itching is often the first sign of infection and begins within one week after close physical contact with an infected partner. If you've had crabs before, you are already sensitized and the itch begins almost immediately.

SCABIES: Itching, which is generally worse at night, often begins within one week after close physical contact with an infected partner. If you have already been sensitized, itching may begin immediately.

SYPHILIS: A chancre, or painless red ulcer, appears on your penis or anal region within ninety days after sex with an infected partner (average two to four weeks). If untreated, the chancre heals but the disease advances.